HOW TO READ AN ECG

FOURTH EDITION

WITHDRAWN

Margaret G. Blowers, RN, BSN

Roberta Smith Sims, RN, MEd

D1297103

Delmar Publishers Inc.®
Albany, N.Y. 12212

Medical Economics Books
Oradell, N.J. 07649

Publisher of this printing:

Delmar Publishers Inc.
2 Computer Drive West
Box 15-015
Albany, New York 12212

Executive Editor: Susan L. Newkirk

ISBN: 0-8273-3697-7

Library of Congress Cataloging-in-Publication Data

Blowers, Margaret G.
How to read an ECG.

Includes index.
1. Electrocardiography.   2. Cardiovascular disease nursing. I. Sims, Roberta Smith. II. Title.
[DNLM: 1. Electrocardiography. WG 140 B657h] RC683.5.E5B59 1988
616.1′ 207547   ISBN 0-87489-497-2   87-28185

Medical Economics Company Inc.
Oradell, New Jersey 07649

First Edition	May 1973
Second Edition	June 1977
Third Edition	October 1983
Fourth Edition	May 1988

Printed in the United States of America

CONTENTS

PART I

PART II

PART III

PART IV

PART V

PUBLISHER'S NOTES

How to Read an ECG originated as a three-part series by Herbert H. Butler, MD, in the January, February, and March 1973, issues of RN Magazine. Compiled in book form for convenient reference, it quickly became a bestseller, used extensively in nursing schools, hospital in-service training programs, and AMA seminars. In June 1977, a revised edition was published, updated and greatly expanded by Margaret Blowers and Roberta Smith (now Sims).

This fourth edition which continues to emphasize the concise, straightforward approach of the first three editions, has been revised and expanded to include more information on application of the 12-lead ECG and other parameters for evaluation of the patient. Treatment modalities for the various rhythm disturbances have been updated. The pacemaker section has been amplified. Differentiation of rhythm problems from the ventricles is augmented by further examples. A brief quiz for each part has been added to reinforce the learner's comprehension.

Margaret G. Blowers, RN, BSN, is an instructor in intensive cardiac and respiratory nursing care for the Nursing Education Department of Hackensack Medical Center, Hackensack, NJ. She is a graduate of the Frances Payne Bolton School of Nursing of Case Western Reserve University in Cleveland, Ohio, and of Seton Hall University in South Orange, N.J.

Roberta Smith Sims, RN, MEd, is coordinator of the Practical Nursing Program at Warren County Technical School, Washington, NJ. She was previously an instructor in cardiac care and ECG and arrhythmias. She is a graduate of St. Luke's Hospital Nursing School, Bethlehem, PA; Cedar Crest College, Allentown, PA; and Lehigh University, Bethlehem, PA.

The table on the inside front cover, "Determining Heart Rate," is reprinted from Haddad A, Dean DC: *Interpreting ECGs: An Advanced Self-Test Guide,* Oradell, NJ: Medical Economics Company, 1981. The cross-section view of an electrode on page 2 is reproduced from Buchsbaum WH, Goldsmith B: *Electrical Safety in the Hospital,* Oradell, NJ: Medical Economics Company.

This book has been designed for use as a stand-up flip chart. See the instructions printed on the flap of the inside back cover.

INTRODUCTION

Thousands of heart patients are being saved in hospitals today because of prompt assessment and treatment of cardiac arrhythmias by nurses and other trained emergency personnel. Usually it is the nurse who is at the patient's side when a cardiac catastrophe occurs, and it is the nurse who has been largely responsible for the marked decrease in cardiac mortality in coronary- and intensive-care units.

Since lethal arrhythmias also occur outside critical-care units, all healthcare workers—physicians, nurses, paramedics, cardiac-care technicians, ambulance attendants, and so on—as well as police, firefighters, and other emergency personnel can use some basic knowledge of ECGs. At the very least, they should be able to recognize the most dangerous cardiac abnormalities. Recognition of a dangerous arrhythmia—particularly through alert observation of an abnormal ECG—can considerably improve a patient's chance for survival.

The book focuses on the basic knowledge needed concerning (1) the use of electrocardiographic monitors, (2) ECG fundamentals and other means of assessing the effects of cardiac dysfunction in the patient, (3) noncatastropic supraventricular arrhythmia analysis, (4) life-threatening ventricular arrhythmias and conduction problems, (5) miscellaneous rhythm disturbances, and (6) a self-test.

This book is most useful as a primer or simplified orientation to ECG monitoring for medical students, nurses, or the various allied health disciplines that now work with patients in situations where cardiac monitoring is used. Radiology technicians, respiratory and physical therapists, as well as emergency personnel and medical office assistants will be finding ever more use of ECG monitoring in the workplace. The efficacy of this expanding method of patient protection is directly dependent on people trained to recognize and respond to the usual cause of sudden cardiac death—arrhythmias.

Treatment must always be based on a combination of comprehensive knowledge of the effects of arrhythmias, clinical information about the individual patients' condition, and awareness of legal limitations imposed by the institution or local government.

GLOSSARY

Aberrant   Wandering from the normal course.

Antiarrhythmia drugs   Those commonly administered to counteract irregularities in cardiac rate or rhythm.

Arrhythmia   A cardiac rhythm disturbance due to a dysfunction in impulse formation or conduction.

Artifact   Lines displayed on the ECG tracing which are not caused by the electrical impulses of the heart.

Atrium (pl. **atria**)   The upper chambers of the heart which receive the return flow of venous blood.

Automaticity   The ability of the myocardial cells to discharge an electrical impulse.

Bundle of His   Small band of cardiac muscle fibers that disperses the atrial contraction consistently to the ventricles.

Cardiac arrest   Ventricular standstill. The heart stops beating and death can occur in one to three minutes.

Cardiac output   The amount of blood pumped by the heart per minute (cardiac output = Heart rate x Stroke volume).

Cardioversion   An electric shock, synchronized with the QRS complex or ventricular beat, that depolarizes the entire heart in order to allow the SA node to resume control.

Compensatory mechanism   Ability of the heart to change rate and rhythm in order to maintain adequate cardiac output.

Coronary arteries   Small vessels that originate from the aorta above the aortic valve and provide the blood supply to the heart.

Defibrillation   Electrical shock not timed to the cardiac cycle. It depolarizes all fibrillating myocardial cells simultaneously, allowing the SA node to resume pacing.

Depolarization   Process by which the impulse from the SA node stimulates the change of chemicals through the cell membrane. This reverses the electrical polarity of the myocardial cell.

Diastole   Resting and filling phase of the cardiac cycle.

Dissociation   Separate rhythms in different parts of the heart.

Dysrhythmia   A cardiac rhythm disturbance. In the context of this text, may be used interchangeably with the term arrhythmia.

Ectopic beat   One arising from a focus outside the sinus node.

Electrocardiogram (ECG)   A graphic recording of the electrical activity produced by the heart muscle.

Electrodes   Contacts applied to designated points on a patient's limbs or chest wall. They transmit the heart's electrical impulses to a graphic recorder.

Escape beat   One that arises from the junctional or ventricular tissue after a prolonged pause with no beats occurring.

Exit block   A type of conduction disturbance in which the impulse does not leave the place of origin.

Extrasystole   Systole originating outside the sinus node; a premature beat is usually an extrasystole.

Fibrillation   Arrhythmia characterized by disorganized electrical activity with erratic quivering of the heart muscle instead of a contraction of the chamber.

Ischemia   Deficiency of blood supply to tissue because of arterial constriction or obstruction.

Isoelectric   Neither negative nor positive in electrical potential; giving off no current, producing a straight line on the ECG.

Myocardial infarction   Death of an area of cardiac muscle tissue due to inadequate blood oxygen supply.

Pacemaker (physiological)   Normally the SA node, which sends out regular impulses to stimulate the myocardium.

Pacemaker artifact   (blip or spike) The ECG waveform produced by a mechanical pacemaker impulse. It can be either an upward or a downward deflection depending on how the pacing wires are connected to the pulse generator.

Parasympathetic nervous system   Portion of autonomic system that acts to maintain a slow heart rate. The vagus nerve is the heart's connection for this system.

PAT   Paroxysmal atrial tachycardia.

Precordial ECG waves   Those emanating from chest leads of a 12-lead ECG.

Pre-excitation   Premature activation of a portion of the ventricle.

P wave   The ECG representation of the electrical impulse going through the atria.

PVC   Premature ventricular contraction. Also called PVB (beat), PVD (depolarization), VPC, or VPB.

QRS complex   The letters have no specific meaning; Q, R, and S waves represent the electrical impulse going through the ventricles.

Re-entry   An arrhythmia mechanism by which an impulse is conducted in one direction and returns through another pathway (echo beat). If this reactivates the earlier site, rapid repetitive firing occurs.

Refractory   Not responsive to stimuli or treatment.

Repolarization   Return of electrical potential to the normal (resting) state.

SA (sinoatrial) node   The normal physiological pacemaker in the heart.

Sensing   The mechanical ability of the artificial pacemaker to detect a natural contraction.

Sequential pacing (dual chamber pacing) The use of two electrodes to pace the atria and then the ventricles in a way that approximates the normal heart cycle.

Sick sinus syndrome A failing sinus node, manifested as severe slowing, blocking, or arresting of the SA node, or as an alternating sinus tachycardia-sinus bradycardia pattern.

Supraventricular tachycardia (SVT) A general term for a rhythm disturbance that originates from the Bundle of His or above the ventricles.

Sympathetic nervous system Portion of autonomic nervous system that acts to increase the heart rate.

Systole Contraction phase of the cardiac cycle.

Threshold The minimum amount of energy (measured in milliamperes) on an artificial pacemaker that is sufficient to produce a contraction.

Vector An electrical force of known magnitude and direction.

Ventricles The thick-walled, muscular lower chambers of the heart.

Vulnerable period The time during the cardiac cycle when the ventricular cells are partially repolarized, but not completely ready for normal response. This occurs during the T wave. Stimulation at this time may produce an erractic rhythm response.

HOW TO READ AN ECG

PART 1

Electrocardiographic monitoring
Types of monitoring equipment
Troubleshooting monitoring problems
Electrical safety

Electrocardiographic monitoring

Electrocardiographic monitoring provides a means of continuous observation of the electrical activity of the heart. In hospital monitoring systems, the oscilloscopic viewing screen is the primary form of display device used. Continuous monitoring can be used to determine conduction of impulses and irritability of tissue as well as to detect alterations in rate and rhythm. Changes in the ECG also indicate the effects of drugs and electrolytes and areas of damage to the myocardium.

Electrode application. The heart is activated by electrical impulses conducted through specialized myocardial tissue. Electrodes are metal contacts that sense the electrical activity of the heart at the body's surface and conduct it to a monitor or electrocardiograph. Most monitoring electrodes are the disposable, floating disc type.

In special circumstances, metal plate or needle electrodes may be used. Suction cup electrodes are usually applied to record a 12-lead ECG.

Normally, the skin offers resistance to the passage of the heart's electrical impulses. To improve conduction, the electrode application sites are shaved

Cross-section of disposable, self-adhesive electrode

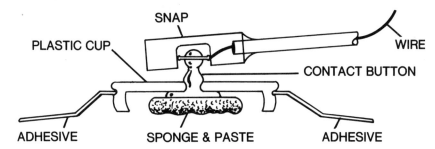

and cleansed with alcohol. Then the skin is dried with a brisk rub. Some protocols recommend mild abrasion or other special skin preparation. Follow the recommended procedures for your system.

Before applying a disposable electrode, check to see that the gelled pad is moist. Then attach the electrode using finger pressure around the adhesive surface.

Each electrode is attached to a lead wire with a snap or clip-on fastener. Depending on the system, two to five lead wires are jacked into a patient cable that acts as an extension cord to the monitor.

Lead placement. The choice of a lead is determined by monitoring needs and institutional protocol. While it is possible to place electrodes in various locations to obtain a tracing, only consistent placement will provide a standard for comparison. To reduce artifact, avoid placing electrodes over bony protuberances, large muscle masses, or skin lesions.

The bipolar system consists of a negative (RA or right arm) electrode, a positive (LA or left arm) electrode, and a third electrode (G or ground) that reduces artifact for a clearer picture. The following diagrams show two common electrode placement schemes for continuous monitoring using the three-electrode system.

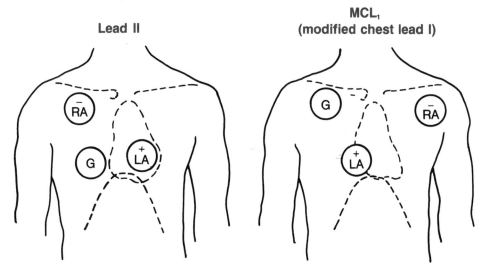

Lead II

MCL₁
(modified chest lead I)

A five-electrode system with a multiple-lead selector is capable of showing cardiac conduction from many viewpoints.

Types of monitoring equipment

Monitoring equipment varies in complexity and capability. The information that follows may apply more to some types of equipment than to others. Refer to the manufacturer's operating instructions for specific information about your machine.

Controls. The ECG monitor is activated by an on-off switch. Other controls enhance observation and provide alarms in cases of unstable heart rhythms.

The height of the upward deflections can be regulated by a knob labeled "gain," "size" or "sensitivity." With a typical unit, the gain should be turned up until the beeper or QRS light is activated with each spike or beat. Then the control should be set slightly above the threshold point to ensure consistent triggering. A 1-millivolt button is used to standardize the gain for a 12-lead ECG. The position control is used to raise or lower the ECG tracing on the display screen.

The rate number displayed by most monitoring systems is an indicator of the number of beats sensed, but it is not an adequate substitute for a pulse check. Adjustable low- and high-rate alarms should be set at the points where a rate change would cause a significant reduction in cardiac output. It is usually desirable to be alerted if the rate drops below 50 beats per minute or increases 30 beats per minute above a normal rate.

With oscilloscopic display systems, the 25/50-mm sweep indicator regulates the speed of the image moving across the screen. The standard is 25 mm or 1 inch per second, but the 50-mm setting spreads out the waveforms for closer observation. Always label any tracings recorded on chart paper at the 50-mm setting, and return the setting to standard afterwards. Some monitors have a "freeze" button to stop the moving image on the screen. An outlet for a jack to synchronize a defibrillator may be located on the front or back of the machine.

Sophisticated systems may have screens with several channels to display other hemodynamic measurements. If these lines are not being used, they may be converted into a longer, continuous ECG tracing for a "cascade" effect.

Monitors with an "INOP" or "LEAD FAULT" signal distinguish between a patient problem and a mechanical problem or defective electrode/cable connection.

The **central station** of a typical monitoring system consists of a multichannel oscilloscope for continuous viewing of a number of rhythms simultaneously, an alarm system, and a recorder or write-out device. Recorders with date-time indicators can be turned on manually or may be activated

automatically when an alarm sounds or a major arrhythmia occurs. A system with a memory unit stores information for a time so that complexes can be retrieved for analysis.

Computerized systems. The addition of computers or automated systems enhances the probability of catching the occasional or subtle dysrhythmia. The computer senses minute changes in configuration and rhythm and provides continuous observation and data.

The computer first "learns" the patient's normal beat. Complexes that are wider and occur prematurely will be registered as ventricular premature beats. Premature beats with "normal" QRS configurations are recorded as supraventricular. When programmed to detect pacemaker beats, the computer scans for and registers the combined pacemaker artifact (blip) and wide complex as a paced beat.

As the findings of the computer are verified or questioned by the nurse or technician, a greater degree of accuracy can be obtained. Histories of ECG and other events are often available for the last minute, hour, 12-hour span, etc. Trends in the patient's status can be seen and the effect of medication and treatment evaluated.

Telemetry is a method for transmitting electrocardiographic signals via radio waves. Signals are relayed from patients in various areas of a hospital to a central receiving station. They are then wired into a monitor for oscilloscopic display and/or printout.

When telemetry is used, the ECG electrodes are connected to a pocket-size, battery-operated transmitter worn by the patient, who can be ambulatory within a defined sending area. Telemetry transmitters can impair the performance of some demand pacemakers. Consult the operating manuals of the specific telemetry unit and pacemaker for details.

Telemetry is also used by emergency personnel in the field, who connect the patient electrodes to a more powerful transmitter that relays signals to a hospital receiving unit. Physicians can then observe rhythms and order appropriate therapy.

Some hospitals and diagnostic centers also use radio waves or telephone lines to transmit ECG signals to outside computer centers for immediate interpretation.

Portable Holter monitoring systems record a continuous ECG during the course of a patient's daily activities. Electrodes are attached to a recorder that is worn on a shoulder strap or belt. During the test period, which may last as long as 24 hours, the outpatient keeps a running record of all his activities and symptoms.

The system is used to document transient and/or asymptomatic arrhythmias, to correlate ECG changes with exertion, stress, or symptoms, and to evaluate antiarrhythmic drug therapy.

Portable monitor-defibrillator units, designed for emergency use, can give a "quick look" picture when the operator places the electrode paddles directly on the chest. To provide an image similar to lead II, the negative paddle is placed over the upper chest to the right of the sternum and the positive paddle is placed over the lower left chest. Conduction gel or saline pads improve the picture and permit immediate use of the paddles for defibrillation if indicated.

These portable units are used both in the field by paramedics and for emergency resuscitation in hospitals or other medical settings. The monitor portion of the unit can be detached to accompany a patient during transport.

Note: Battery-operated monitors function for a relatively short period of time. Consult the operating manual for limitations on your model. Be sure the unit is fully charged before transport.

Troubleshooting monitoring problems

Artifacts are distortions of the ECG waveform resulting from extraneous electrical or mechanical activity that is not part of the natural impulse. These distortions can make accurate interpretation difficult.

Whenever there is a disturbance or change in the tracing, check the patient. If the patient is stable, look at the equipment. Poor electrode contact is the most frequent cause of unwanted artifact.

The following guide can help you troubleshoot common monitoring problems:

Tracing shows:

Check for and correct:

1. straight line
   - attachment of lead wire to wrong cable outlet
   - gain set too low
   - lead selector switch at wrong setting
   - detached lead

2. loss of signal (intermittent or continuous)
   - loose electrode
   - break in connection anywhere from lead wire to wall plug
   - static electricity, especially with low humidity
   - barriers to transmission with telemetry

Intermittent loss of signal

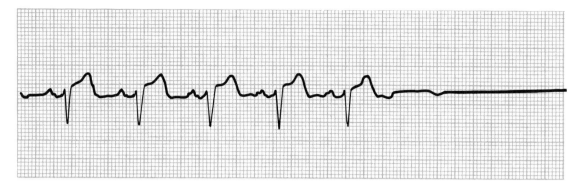

Tracing shows:
3. wide baseline
(60-cycle or alternating current interference)

Check for and correct:
- inadequate grounding
- broken or damaged wires on patient cable or three-prong plugs
- patient cable lying parallel with any other power cord
- high-voltage source or other electrical activity nearby, or on same circuit
- electrical defect in any adjacent equipment

Wide baseline from 60-cycle interference

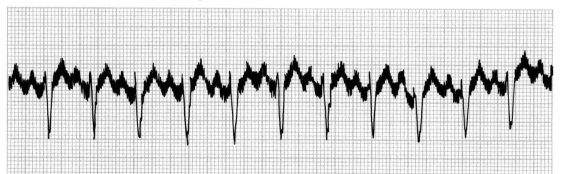

Tracing shows:
4. wandering baseline

Check for and correct:
- loose electrodes
- poor skin prep
- body movement
- dried or lost electrode gel
- patient cable not secured
- electrode placement sensing respiratory movement

Tracing shows:	**Check for and correct:**
5. multiple irregular spikes between QRS complexes	• patient movement, shivering, nervous tension, muscle tremor, respiratory activity, or seizures
	• stretch or strain on leads or patient cable
	• loose or dry electrodes
	• electrodes placed over bony prominences or areas of high muscle activity

Multiple irregular spikes and wandering baseline

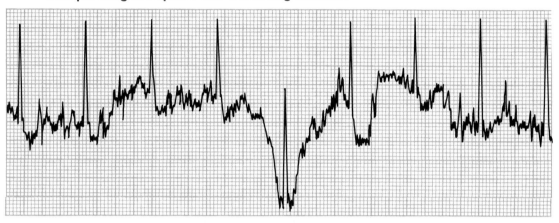

False or inappropriate alarms can be minimized by checking the following:

Problem:	**Check for and correct:**
1. false high-rate alarms	• monitor gain set too high—Ps or Ts are being registered as QRS spikes, especially with MCL$_1$ (modified chest lead I) setting
	• high T wave from possible hyperkalemia
	• high-rate alarm setting does not allow for normal patient motion
	• patient is restless, cold, tense, etc., causing artifacts that are sensed as extra beats
2. false low-rate alarms	• gain set too low—some QRS spikes are not sensed
	• low-amplitude QRS from lead placement or cardiac pathology
	• electrodes placed less than 3 inches apart

Electrical safety

Conditions causing alternating current (AC) interference on the ECG tracing may be symptoms of a possible electrical hazard. Remember that the body can be a conductor of electricity. Intravenous or arterial lines and especially pacing wires bypass the skin's normal resistance and can conduct current into the heart. Even small amounts of current can cause fibrillation when delivered directly to the myocardium.

Patients in critical-care areas who are connected to various machines and tubes are potentially vulnerable to electrical accidents. Observe the following precautions:

1. Handle equipment carefully. Protect cords from heat, alcohol, and traffic pathways.
2. Use only equipment with intact three-prong plugs. Do not use "cheaters" (three-prong to two-prong adapting plugs).
3. Do not use damaged plugs, frayed wires, or outlets that will not firmly hold a plug.
4. Never remove a plug by pulling on the cord.
5. Report and immediately discontinue use of any equipment that emits a shock or tingle.
6. Do not permit your body to be a pathway to ground by touching two electrical devices or a patient catheter and an electrical device simultaneously.
7. Wear rubber gloves when handling exposed parts of a pacing catheter or when changing dressings. Keep all pacemaker connections insulated.
8. Whenever possible, if two electrical devices are used with one patient, connect them to the same wall outlet cluster.
9. Never plug in or switch on electrical equipment while touching pathways to ground (metal bedrails, plumbing, etc.).
10. Make sure that no one is touching any part of the patient or bed during cardioversion or defibrillation.

All electrical equipment used in providing patient care should be checked at regular intervals in accordance with the most recent standards for hospital accreditation.

HOW TO READ AN ECG

PART II

Normal ECG and related heart anatomy
The ECG leads and the 12-lead ECG
Identification of MI and diagnostic tests
Assessing effects of arrhythmias

Normal ECG and related heart anatomy

The electrocardiogram presents a visible record of the heart's electrical activity by means of a stylus that traces the activity on a continuously moving strip of special paper.

Normal ECG

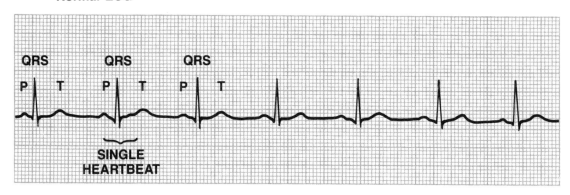

Normal ECG. All beats appear as a similar pattern, equally spaced, and have three major units: P wave, QRS complex, and T wave.

Normal single heartbeat

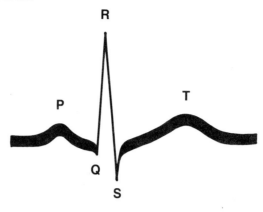

Normal single heartbeat. Each beat manifests as five major waves: P, Q, R, S, and T. The Q, R, and S all represent the same part of the heart (ventricles). They are usually referred to as a unit: the QRS complex.

The heart in relation to the ECG

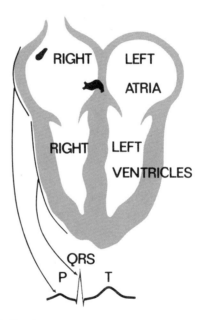

The heart in relation to the ECG. Each wave represents transmission of an electrical impulse through the heart muscle (depolarization), which causes the muscle to contract and thus eject blood. The P wave reflects the impulse going through the atria. The QRS complex reflects the impulse going through the ventricles. The T wave is produced by the electrical recovery (repolarization) of the ventricles.

Depolarization. As the electrical impulse moves across the cells of the myocardium, the polarity (negative or positive electrical charge) of the cells is changed.

The resting cell has a negative charge: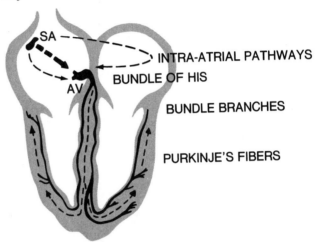

The electrical impulse carries a positive charge into the cell, changing the polarity:

This is called depolarization:

It is followed by a continuing wave of repolarization that restores the cell to its original charge:

The cell is then ready to receive another stimulus.

Normal electrical pathway

SA

INTRA-ATRIAL PATHWAYS

BUNDLE OF HIS

AV

BUNDLE BRANCHES

PURKINJE'S FIBERS

Normal electrical pathway. The impulse is conducted to the muscle cells by way of specialized tissue that has automaticity and conductivity. All myocardial tissue has these properties, but they are developed to a greater degree in the conduction system.

The electrical impulse originates in the sinoatrial (SA) node—the normal physiological pacemaker—located near the top of the right atrium. The impulse spreads through intra-atrial pathways to the atrioventricular (AV) node located at the junction of the atria and ventricles. After a brief delay, the impulse continues through the bundle of His, the right and left bundle branches, and Purkinje fibers, and finally activates the ventricular muscle cells. Both the SA and AV nodes are innervated by the sympathetic system, which increases the heart rate, and by the parasympathetic system (vagus nerve), which slows the rate.

The SA node normally discharges impulses at a rate of 60–100 times per minute, AV junctional tissue at 40–60, and Purkinje fibers at 20–40. The pacemaker firing at the fastest rate controls the heartbeat. The presence of

multiple pacemakers provides a reserve or backup system against cardiac arrest.

ECG paper

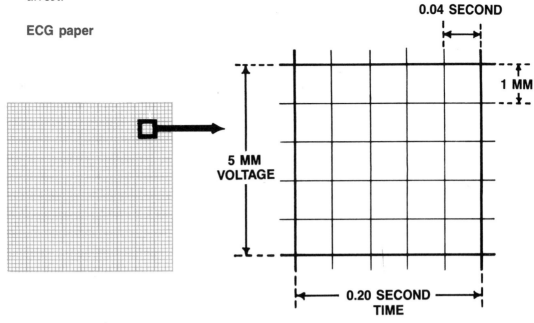

ECG paper. To understand the significance of each wave and interval, we need to know the significance of the small and large blocks on the ECG paper. The paper moves through the ECG machine at the rate of 1 inch per second (standard setting). One small block represents 0.04 second on the horizontal line and 1 mm on the vertical line. Since a large block is five small blocks wide and five high, each large block represents 0.20 second (horizontal) and 5 mm (vertical). 10 mm = 1 millivolt of electrical activity.

Now that we know these basic measurements and are familiar with the relation of the ECG waves to the heart anatomy, let's discuss the significance of each wave and interval:

P wave

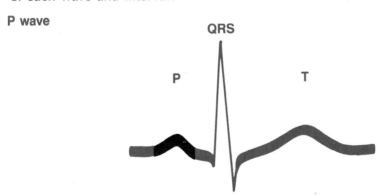

The **P wave** is the first upward deflection and represents the atrial depolarization. Enlargement of the P wave might occur in such conditions as mitral

stenosis or chronic obstructive pulmonary disease, which would cause atrial hypertrophy. The P wave is usually considered enlarged if it is more than three small blocks (3 mm) high and/or three small blocks (0.12 second) wide.

PR interval

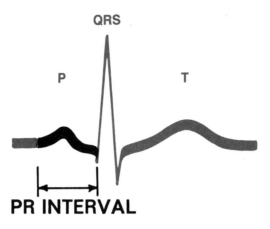

The **PR interval** extends from the beginning of the P wave to the onset of the QRS. It represents conduction of the impulse through the atria and the AV node. The PR interval is abnormally lengthened when the impulse is forced to travel at a slower rate, which can occur in arteriosclerosis, inflammation, insufficient oxygen supply, or scarring from rheumatic heart disease. It can also occur as an effect of depressant drugs or digitalis. The normal PR interval is three to five small blocks wide (0.12–0.20 second).

QRS complex

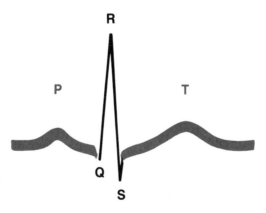

The **QRS complex** consists of three deflections: Q wave, the downstroke before the R; R wave, the first upward deflection; and S wave, the downstroke following the R wave. Not every QRS complex shows a discrete Q, R, and S wave, but the configuration is still referred to as the QRS complex to denote a ventricular impulse. An enlarged Q wave (over a small

square wide or greater in depth than one-third the height of the QRS) may indicate a myocardial infarction. A vertically enlarged R wave usually indicates enlarged ventricles. The normal duration of the QRS is two and one-half small squares or less (0.10 second).

ST segment

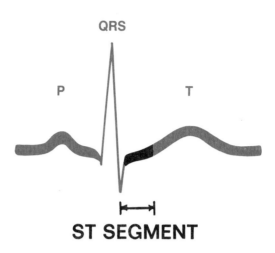

ST SEGMENT

The **ST segment** begins at the end of the S wave (the point where the line turns right) and ends at the beginning of the T wave. It is elevated in an acute myocardial infarction or muscle injury. It is depressed when the heart muscle isn't getting a sufficient supply of oxygen—for example, during an episode of angina or coronary insufficiency. It may sag as an effect of digitalis. ST changes are usually transient.

T wave

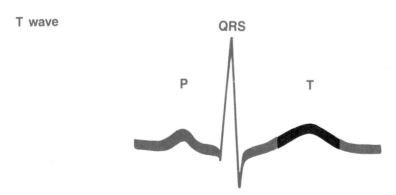

The **T wave** represents electrical recovery of the ventricular contraction. (The electrons are in the process of moving back into the normal resting position.) The T wave is flat or inverted in response to ischemia, position change, food intake, or certain drugs. It may be elevated when the serum potassium is elevated. The normal T wave is no more than 10 small blocks (10 mm) high in the precordial (chest) leads and five small blocks (5 mm) high in the remaining leads.

U wave
QT interval

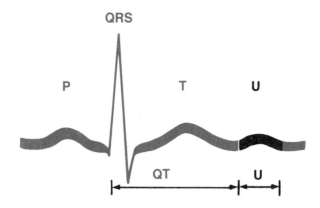

The **U wave** is a small upward deflection following the T wave. It is seldom present, but may occur when the serum potassium level is low.

The **QT interval** represents the time from the beginning of the Q wave (downward deflection following the P wave) through the QRS and the T wave. It includes the time until the T wave is completed (goes back to the baseline). The time of this interval should be less than one-half of the R-R interval (from the peak of one R wave to the peak of the next R wave). If the QT time is prolonged, it presents an extended opportunity for stray irritable impulses to excite the heart tissue and trigger dangerous ventricular rhythms. After the T wave is completed the tissue is repolarized and at rest, ready to respond normally. Impulses that arrive during the T wave find the ventricular tissue incompletely recovered and vulnerable to an erratic response. Certain drugs, such as quinidine, procainamide hydrochloride (Pronestyl) and disopyramide phosphate (Norpace) can prolong the QT interval and thus predispose to ventricular tachycardia. If a patient is receiving the drugs named, the QT interval should be measured, and drugs and electrolytes regulated to maintain normal function.

The ECG leads

ECG leads are formed by placing electrodes at specific places on the body and amplifying and recording the electrical activity that occurs along this pathway. A vector is a force of a known magnitude and direction. The recordings may be said to display certain vectors or electrical forces traveling in the direction between the leads.

The first three bipolar leads used by ECG pioneer Dr. Einthoven were leads I, II, and III recording the electrical activity along the pathway from a negative electrode toward a relatively positive electrical pole. (Electricity flows only when there is a difference in polarity.)

Each lead records the same electrical impulse on the ECG but from a different position in relation to the heart. Each can be read separately, or they can be read in combination.

The limb leads show the current flow from one area of the body toward another. Lead I shows electrical activity from the right arm to the left arm, lead II from right arm to left leg, and lead III from left arm to left leg. The right-leg position is not displayed as part of the flow of current through the heart, as it is used for grounding the system. In the 12-lead ECG, the leads are placed on the limbs. For continuous monitoring, these leads are positioned on the chest in a smaller configuration.

Whenever electrical activity flows from a negative pole toward a positive pole, it causes an upward deflection on the ECG tracing. The lead that will show the tallest upward deflections is the one that is parallel to the actual forces in the body. Lead II is frequently used for monitoring as it is usually parallel to the direction of the electrical activity in the heart, and shows an easily visible P wave. Illustrations in this book are taken from lead II unless otherwise labeled.

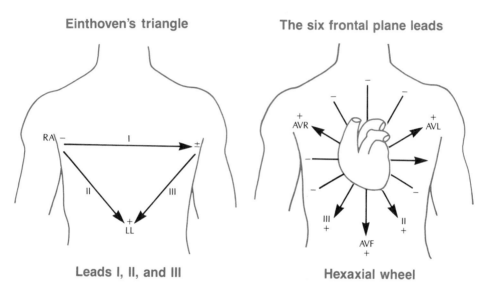

Einthoven's triangle   The six frontal plane leads

Leads I, II, and III   Hexaxial wheel

If more lead placements are used, specific areas of heart dysfunction can be identified. Therefore the positive or exploring electrode is positioned at other sites and by using combinations of other electrodes for the neutral or negative pole, unipolar lead sites are formed.

The abbreviation AVR stands for augmented vector right, an added point of reference for diagnosis. AVL and AVF represent the left-side and left-foot positions, respectively.

The combination of all six leads on the frontal plane gives us a full circle of references to evaluate cardiac function. This is called the hexaxial wheel.

In addition to the frontal plane, a horizontal plane of reference can be used for more precise location of problems.

The **precordial leads** provide points of reference across the chest wall as illustrated. They differentiate right-sided and left-heart events.

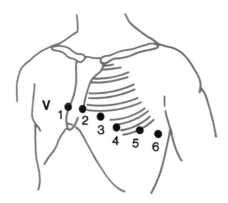

Modified chest lead I (p. 2) is a monitoring lead that simulates precordial lead V_1. This lead will help to differentiate right from left bundle branch block.

To record a routine ECG, 12 leads are used:

On the limbs: I, II, III, AVR, AVL, AVF

On the chest: V_1, V_2, V_3, V_4, V_5, V_6

The same beat can have a different configuration when seen from a different lead. These are the normal variations in the 12-lead ECG.

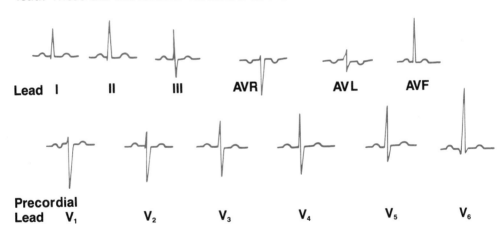

Lead I   **II**   **III**   **AVR**   **AVL**   **AVF**

Precordial Lead V_1   **V_2**   **V_3**   **V_4**   **V_5**   **V_6**

The most important leads to remember in relation to the anatomy of the heart are:

V_1, AVR   Right side of heart

V_2, V_3, V_4 Transition between right and left sides of heart

V_5, V_6, I, AVL   Left side of heart

II, III, AVF   Inferior heart

The area of pathology shown on the ECG can be localized by analyzing tracings from different leads. For example: If an infarct shows up on leads II, III, and AVF only, it is located in the inferior aspect of the heart.

These lead combinations designating specific areas of the heart can be remembered by visualizing them as the positive poles (the arrow ends) shown on the hexaxial wheel, or the areas where the (positive) exploring electrode defines the precordial V leads.

Identification of MI

One of the most significant uses of a 12-lead ECG is to aid in determining whether a myocardial infarction has occurred. The physician can locate the damage by noting which leads show indicative changes. (Leads II, III, and AVF show the inferior or diaphragmatic area of the heart. The precordial or chest leads reflect changes on the anterior surface.) Many factors can influence the 12-lead ECG interpretation. Changes most characteristic of an MI are presented in the following section.

One important point to remember about the ECG interpretation of MI is that about 15 per cent of infarcts show no changes on the initial tracing. ECG changes evolve later in hours or days as tissue damage changes electrical impulse conduction pathways. Therefore, a patient who has symptoms compatible with a heart attack but has a normal ECG should nevertheless be admitted to the hospital for observation, further electrocardiograms, and evaluation. Early treatment may prevent some of the damage that would otherwise occur. Most of the dangerous arrhythmias happen in the very early hours of a heart attack. Monitoring and intervention save many lives.

The usual first finding in an infarct is elevation of the ST segment. This is followed by T wave inversion, which in turn is followed by a large Q wave. As the infarct heals, the Q wave may remain as the only sign of an old infarction. This is the sequence:

Sequence of the ECG following MI

Sequence of the ECG following MI. (1) Normal. (2) Hours after infarction, the ST segment becomes elevated. (3) Hours to days later, the T wave inverts

and the Q wave becomes larger. (4) Days to weeks later, the ST segment returns to near-normal. (5) Weeks to months later, the T wave becomes upright again, but the Q wave may remain large.

Abnormal Q wave

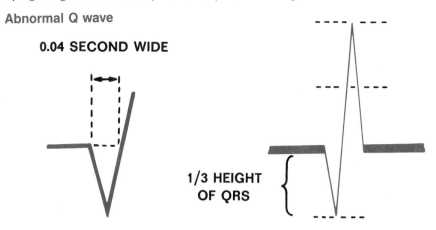

0.04 SECOND WIDE

1/3 HEIGHT OF QRS

Abnormal Q wave. Since a large Q wave is often indicative of an old infarction (except in AVR, where a large Q wave is normal), the question is often asked how large a Q wave can be before it is considered abnormal. A Q wave may be considered abnormal if it is over 0.04 second wide (one small block on the ECG paper), or if it is greater in depth than one-third the height of the QRS complex.

In summary: A fresh myocardial infarction is characterized by ST elevation and T wave inversion. An enlarged Q wave without ST or T wave changes is indicative of an old infarction. No Q wave may appear if the infarction is subendocardial (not through the complete thickness of the wall).

Inferior wall infarction

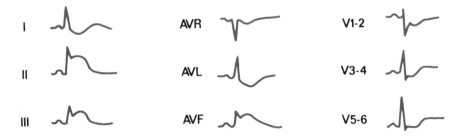

Inferior wall infarction. Very early pattern showing ST elevation in leads II, III, and AVF.

A mirror image of ST depression is seen in opposite leads I, AVL, and precordial leads. This is characteristic of MI and is not seen when ST elevation occurs from other causes such as pericarditis.

Anterior lateral-wall infarction

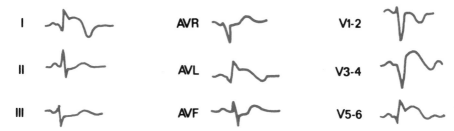

Anterior lateral-wall infarction. A later pattern (many hours to a few days later) shows Q waves and T wave inversion in leads I, AVL, and V$_{4-6}$.

ECG changes in stress testing

An ECG of the resting heart does not predict a myocardial infarction. Unfortunately, some people have shown normal ECGs during a routine physical exam, only to suffer a fatal heart attack shortly thereafter.

An ECG recorded during periods of physical activity may be a more accurate indicator of factors that could predispose to a myocardial infarction. Reason: As the heart rate increases, the myocardium needs more oxygen, and narrow coronary arteries will not provide a sufficient oxygen supply.

Before testing, the candidate is examined by the physician; pertinent cardiopulmonary data, including a resting ECG, are recorded. The patient is stressed by expending measured amounts of energy on a calibrated exercise device such as a treadmill or an ergometer (such as an exercise bicycle). During the activity, a continuous ECG tracing and other vital signs are monitored.

ST depression or elevation indicates myocardial ischemia. Some patients will develop anginal pain during periods of myocardial hypoxia, and others will not. In the presence of typical anginal pain and negative ECG changes, the test is still considered positive. Extra ventricular systoles or other arrhythmias may indicate a positive test.

The following diagram shows some possible ST segment changes under stress:

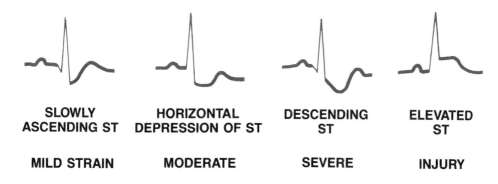

SLOWLY ASCENDING ST	HORIZONTAL DEPRESSION OF ST	DESCENDING ST	ELEVATED ST
MILD STRAIN	MODERATE	SEVERE	INJURY

Other diagnostic tests that can amplify information about the heart include vectorcardiograms, echocardiograms, and phonocardiograms. These noninvasive tests are useful for showing anatomical deviations and functional abnormalities. Radioisotope scans can demonstrate the amount and precise areas of muscle dysfunction. Cardiac catheterization identifies coronary artery patency or obstruction and other abnormalities in blood flow.

Assessing effects of arrhythmias

Whenever there is a change in the ECG during continuous monitoring, assess the patient, and prepare for emergency action if indicated. Record a rhythm strip noting the date and time, and report significant findings. Heart rates below 50 or greater than 140 decrease cardiac output and require prompt attention.

In assessing the effect of the rhythm change, careful observation of the patient will determine the need for treatment and the urgency involved. Evaluate the radial pulse for rate, rhythm, and amplitude, and compare it with the apical pulse rate. A pulse deficit (higher pulse rate at apex) may occur with blocks and atrial tachyarrhythmias. Check for peripheral pulses. If these were previously strong and are now weak or absent, cardiac output is diminished.

Evaluate the blood pressure. A reduced blood pressure may be a warning of congestive heart failure or impending shock. The Mean Arterial Pressure (MAP) is found by adding systolic pressure plus two times diastolic and dividing by three. The MAP should be 60 mmHg or greater for adequate perfusion to the brain and vital organs.

Symptoms such as chest tightness or pain, palpitations, labored or rapid breathing, or inability to breathe lying flat indicate inadequate cardiac oxygenation. Restlessness, confusion, lethargy, personality change, or loss of consciousness can be signs of inadequate oxygen to the brain. Cool, moist skin and pallor suggest reduced blood flow to peripheral areas. Other signs of diminished cardiac function include scant urinary output and/or edema. The patient may complain of feeling weak or tired or have less ability to tolerate physical activity. All these signs of cardiovascular compromise require medical intervention.

Chest auscultation may provide additional information. The presence and level of rales (moist, crackling sounds) in the lungs will help to evaluate the extent of congestive failure. Diffuse rales plus a cough and frothy sputum indicate acute pulmonary edema needing immediate treatment. Changes in heart sounds such as murmurs and friction rubs occur with pathological damage to valves and tissues. More subtle changes requiring a practiced ear accompany some of the dysrhythmias. A third heart sound following the usual "lub dup" is often heard in early congestive failure.

Monitoring other parameters of function can provide more specific

information on the patient's status. Central venous pressure or pulmonary artery pressures can determine the need for fluid reduction or augmentation and offer immediate feedback regarding the efficacy of drug therapy. When cardiac complications such as congestive failure or cardiogenic shock occur, these more precise methods of evaluation are used.

Laboratory information including arterial blood gases for determining respiratory function, electrolytes, drug levels, and serum enzymes can assist in accurate diagnosis. All of these data must be combined with the detailed history and subjective feelings of symptoms the patient describes to plan definitive care. Once a baseline of information is established, a brief update may be sufficient to determine the effect of a rhythm change on the patient's status and the ability to tolerate the rhythm.

HOW TO READ AN ECG

PART III

Format for analyzing arrhythmias
Sinus arrhythmias
Atrial arrhythmias
Junctional (nodal) arrhythmias

Format for analyzing arrhythmias

Summary of normal findings

ECG characteristic	Normal finding
Rhythm	Regular (distance between QRS complexes varies by no more than three small squares)
Rate	60–100 beats per minute (three to five large squares between QRS complexes)
P wave	Present and upright (in leads I, II, AVF, V_2–V_6) All shaped alike
PR interval	P wave precedes QRS Duration greater than three but less than five small squares (0.12–0.20 sec.) Time interval is the same for all beats
QRS complex	Present All shaped alike Duration not more than two and one-half small squares (0.10 sec.)

Normal sinus rhythm

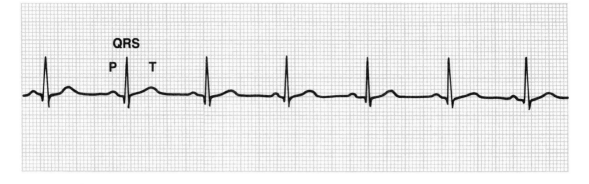

If all findings are normal, **normal sinus rhythm** is present.

Rhythm. Regularity may be determined using calipers or any device that can be marked to show a fixed interval for comparison.

Determining the cardiac rate

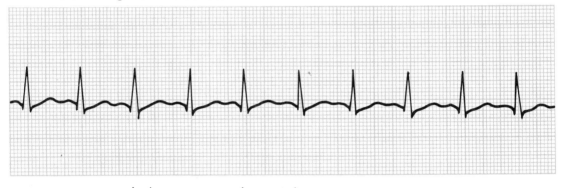

1 LARGE BLOCK   **3 LARGE BLOCKS BETWEEN EACH QRS COMPLEX**

Alternative methods of **determining the cardiac rate. 1.** Since each large block on the ECG paper represents 0.20 second, 300 large blocks represent 1 minute (0.20 × 300 = 60 seconds). If rhythm is regular, count the large blocks between two R waves (QRS complexes) and divide 300 by this figure. In the example above, there are three large blocks between R waves. Dividing 300 by 3 gives us a rate of 100 beats per minute. (If there were two blocks, the rate would be 150; four blocks, 75.) **or: 2.** Count the complexes in a 6-inch strip and multiply by 10 (useful for irregular rhythms). **or: 3.** Use a prepared rate ruler or table (see "Determining Heart Rate" table in the front of the book).

Sinus arrhythmias

Pathway of sinus rhythms. Sinus arrhythmia, sinus tachycardia, and sinus

bradycardia originate in the SA node. The path of their electrical impulses is exactly the same as that of normal sinus rhythm. Because of this, the P wave, the PR interval, and the QRS complex are of normal configuration. The difference lies in the regularity and rate of the impulses.

Sinus arrhythmia

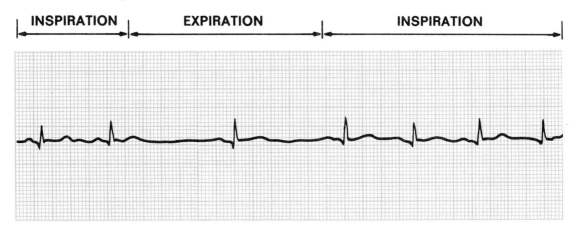

Sinus arrhythmia. All complexes are normal, but the heart rhythm is irregular. The rate increases with inspiration, decreases with expiration. This irregularity is common in children and may occur in adults in relation to certain respiratory patterns. It does not decrease cardiac output and does not lead to more serious arrhythmias.

Sinus tachycardia

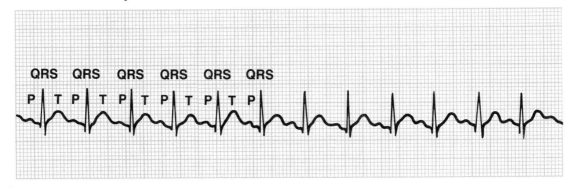

Sinus tachycardia. All complexes are normal, but the heart rate is more than 100. (It seldom exceeds 160.) Excessive sympathetic nerve stimulation causes the increased rate. Common causes are physical activity, anxiety, and fever. An increased rate may also be a compensatory response to decreased cardiac output.

Complications such as congestive heart failure, pulmonary embolism, cardiogenic shock, or bleeding may show sinus tachycardia as an early symptom. Look for the problem. Treatment is directed to the physiologic cause.

25

Sinus bradycardia

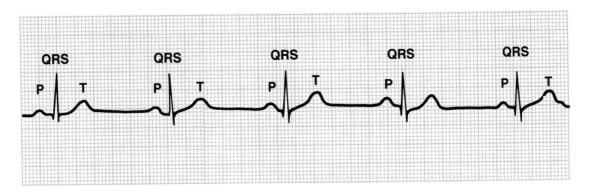

Sinus bradycardia. This arrhythmia is defined as a heart rate below 60 while all complexes remain normal. Sinus bradycardia is seen as an expected manifestation in well-trained athletes. It may occur in patients on digitalis, propranolol (Inderal), morphine, and pressor amines for treatment of low blood pressure. A significant slowing may cause a decrease in cardiac output that can lead to cerebral or coronary insufficiency. An additional hazard is that bradycardia may permit ectopic pacemaker foci to take over, causing serious arrhythmias. Sinus bradycardia may be beneficial in a person at rest but if seen during stress, it could indicate inability of the heart to compensate.

The decision to treat sinus bradycardia is based on an evaluation of the patient's clinical picture. If drug therapy is indicated, IV atropine is used to inhibit the vagus (heart-slowing) nerve, thus speeding up the heart rate. If the patient does not respond, use of an artificial pacemaker may be necessary.

Sinus block

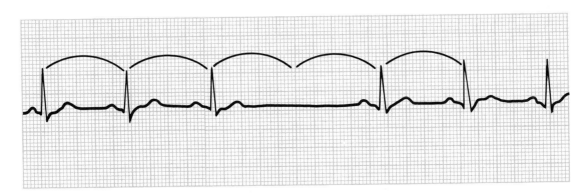

Sinus block occurs when a beat is not transmitted out of the SA node. No P, QRS, or T is present at the cycle interval for one or more beats.

Sinus arrest

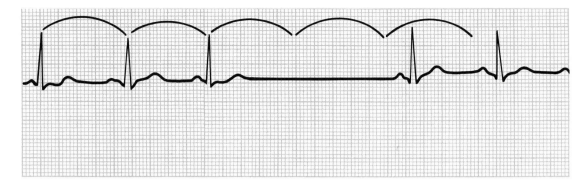

Sinus arrest occurs when the SA node fails to send out an impulse for a period of time. This interval between beats is not a multiple of the heartbeat cycle length.

If either event produces symptoms of hemodynamic insufficiency, treatment (atropine or an artificial pacemaker) is indicated.

Atrial arrhythmias

Portions of atrial tissue may become excitable and initiate impulses. These ectopic foci will control the heartbeat if they occur at a rate faster than impulses from the SA node.

ECG for PAC

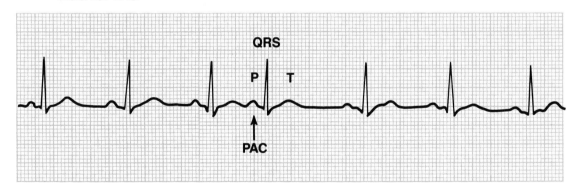

Premature atrial contraction (PAC) is a beat initiated by an ectopic atrial focus that appears early in the cycle (before the next expected sinus beat). Since the impulse arises from a site other than the sinus node, the shape of the P wave and the length of the PR interval may be different. The premature P wave is sometimes difficult to distinguish when it is superimposed on the preceding T wave.

The PAC is usually conducted through the ventricular pathway in the normal manner not affecting the shape of the QRS. A pause will follow the

beat, and the SA node will start a new cycle of sinus beats.

The significance of PACs is that they indicate atrial irritability. Frequent PACs may be warnings of more serious atrial arrhythmias and may be treated. Quinidine is often the drug of choice.

ECG for PAT

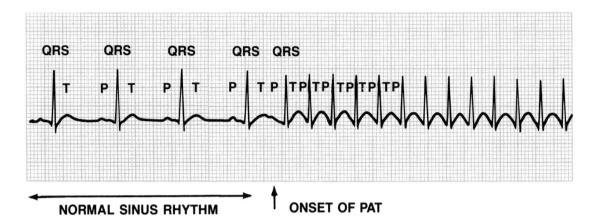

NORMAL SINUS RHYTHM   ONSET OF PAT

Paroxysmal atrial tachycardia (PAT) is an abrupt episode of tachycardia with the heart rate usually between 140 and 250 beats per minute, averaging about 170. The pacemaker site is an ectopic atrial focus. As with a PAC, the P wave may be abnormally shaped, or not seen because it is buried in the preceding T wave. The QRS appears normal.

PAT may be seen in young adults with normal hearts or in individuals with organic disease. The patient frequently complains of a sudden pounding or fluttering in the chest associated with weakness or breathlessness.

The fast rate stresses the heart and increases its need for oxygen. Tachycardia may also diminish cardiac output because of shortened ventricular filling time. The heart is beating so rapidly that the ventricle does not have time to fill completely. Therefore, each beat pumps out less blood. In a relatively asymptomatic and stable patient, sedation and calming measures may be helpful. If PAT persists, the usual treatment is stimulation of the vagus nerve, which slows the heart rate. The physician may accomplish this by carotid sinus massage. Since this can produce dangerous slowing or cardiac arrest, the patient should be monitored, resuscitation equipment should be readily available and an IV line established.

Other measures that stimulate the vagus nerve include: vomiting, stimulating the anal sphincter with a rectal thermometer or tube, and applying pressure to the eyeball. These measures are not suggested as therapy but explain some cardiac responses to such activities. A cough or Valsalva maneuver will increase intrathoracic pressure, decrease venous return, raise the blood pressure, and possibly slow the pulse. A Valsalva maneuver consists of tightening abdominal muscles while holding the breath. This is

similar to the activity of bowel elimination and causes indirect vagal stimulation.

When medication is used to treat atrial tachycardia, IV verapamil (Calan, Isoptin) breaks up the repetitive triggering of impulses. Other drugs, given in a slow IV drip, may be used to provide a vasopressor (and pulse-slowing) effect in patients who are not hypertensive. They are edrophonium (Tensilon) or metaraminol (Aramine). Occasionally, propranolol (Inderal) may be used to slow the heart rate.

When the heart continues to beat rapidly for a period of time, or if the patient becomes symptomatic, a synchronized electrical shock (cardioversion) can be used for immediate conversion.

ECG for ATRIAL TACHYCARDIA WITH BLOCK (or PAT with block)

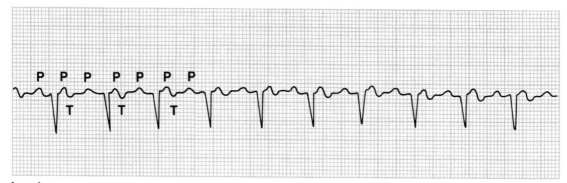

Lead MCL₁ Most cases of PAT exhibit no block, and all the impulses are transmitted by the AV node to the ventricles. Occasionally, some beats are not conducted to the ventricles—a condition called **PAT with block.** The atrial rate is 140–250, and the ventricular rate is slower. This is frequently seen as a result of digitalis toxicity. The block may be regular or irregular.

Re-entry. Many rapid atrial arrhythmias are caused by a re-entry mechanism. Re-entry is a conduction disturbance in which an impulse travels through an area and returns through another pathway to reactivate the original area. It can occur because of conduction problems or disturbances in the refractory period. Every time an impulse travels around the circuit, it triggers another beat. Re-entry may be seen as a single premature beat (echo beat) or in a pattern of repetitive impulses (circus movement).

Atrial flutter is a rapid, regular firing of an irritable ectopic focus in the atrium. It is probably due to a re-entry mechanism. It usually occurs in a pathologic (arteriosclerotic or rheumatic) heart, in contrast to PAT, which may be associated with a normal heart.

The flutter ("F") waves take on a saw-toothed appearance because they are coming from a focus other than the sinus node at a very rapid rate. The atrial rate is between 250 and 350 impulses per minute. Not all of the impulses are

conducted, so the ventricular rate is usually slower. The ventricular response may be regular or irregular.

Note these differences to identify types of supraventricular tachycardia:

1. The atrial rate in sinus tachycardia goes up gradually to 150/minute.
2. The atrial rate in PAT is 140–250/minute and starts abruptly.
3. The atrial rate in atrial flutter is 250–350/minute.

ECG for atrial flutter

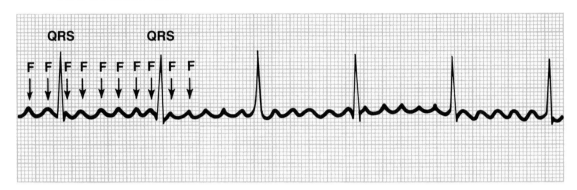

ECG for atrial flutter. The arrows indicate the F waves that are coming from the fast ectopic focus in the atrium. Notice that not every wave stimulates a QRS complex. Since the abnormality is above the AV node, the QRS complexes that appear are normal in configuration.

Because the impulses are coming so rapidly, the AV node cannot accept and conduct each one, and therefore some degree of blockage occurs at the node. For example: If the atrial rate is 300, the ventricular rate (same as the pulse rate) may be 150. The block is thus said to be 2:1, since there are two atrial impulses per one ventricular response. In the diagram, five or six F waves precede each QRS.

Treatment of atrial flutter is indicated if the ventricular rate is sufficiently rapid to be potentially dangerous to the patient.

A fast cardiac rate is relatively ineffectual and may lead to congestive heart failure. The quickest way to slow a very fast flutter is by elective cardioversion. By using low voltage, depolarization of all heart tissue is accomplished with the electrical energy of the defibrillator paddles. The discharge is synchronized with the QRS to avoid any stimulus occurring during the vulnerable period, the T wave. Cardioversion breaks the re-entry cycle and permits the sinus node to gain control. Before the procedure, the patient is sedated with IV Valium and loses awareness for the event. Verapamil (Calan, Isoptin) or quinidine may be given following the cardioversion to prevent recurrence. IV verapamil may break the re-entry without cardioversion. An alternative treatment by drug therapy may be the use of digitalis to increase the level of AV block, thus slowing the ventricular response, and quinidine to slow the atrial activity. Quinidine alone is not given because as the atrial rate slows, there is a point at which each atrial impulse will be conducted,

resulting in an extremely fast ventricular rate (around 200). This would require immediate cardioversion.

Multifocal atrial tachycardia occurs when many ectopic atrial areas produce impulses. Several P's bombard the AV node before a beat is conducted. Different-shaped P waves and varying PR intervals are characteristic. This is frequently seen in patients with chronic lung disease and may be a harbinger of atrial fibrillation.

Atrial fibrillation is a very fast atrial rate arising from many ectopic foci. There is an irregular ventricular response, normal P waves are replaced by irregular rapid waves, and the total atrial configuration may resemble a wavy baseline or almost straight line.

These waves (often called fibrillatory or "f" waves) assume different shapes because different parts of the atrial tissue are depolarized in a variable, uncoordinated way. This occurs in enlarged atrial chambers often impaired by arteriosclerotic heart disease or scar tissue from surgery or infections such as rheumatic fever. Impulses rebound at various times from this uneven depolarization, producing a quivering action instead of an organized atrial contraction. A significant volume of blood which would have been contributed toward ventricular filling by the atrial "kick"/contraction is lost. The atrial component accounts for 15 to 30 per cent of the cardiac output.

Normal pathway   **Atrial fibrillation pathway**

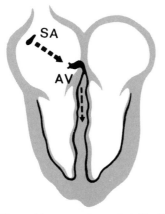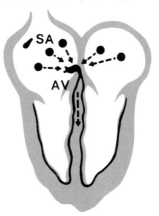

Since P waves in atrial fibrillation are not clearly discernible, the atrial rate cannot be measured but is much faster than the ventricular rate. With no definite P waves, no PR interval can be determined. The ventricular rate may be fast or slow but will be irregular. If it becomes regular, this usually indicates a junctional pacemaker is controlling the ventricles. This is a form of AV dissociation which may result from digitalis toxicity.

The treatment of atrial fibrillation depends on the patient's clinical condition, cardiac rate, and drug status. If atrial fibrillation is a new change and the ventricular rate is very fast, cardioversion may be instituted. Cardioversion may be complicated if the patient is on digitalis, for the drug predisposes the

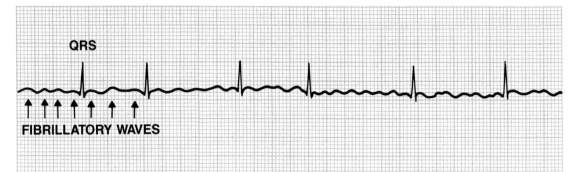

heart to serious arrhythmias after an electrical shock. The risk of arrhythmias increases as the number of watt-seconds is increased. If the patient has been in atrial fibrillation for more than a few days, anticoagulant therapy is instituted before cardioversion is attempted. This is done because clots may form in the fibrillating atria and could be disseminated into the circulation as the atria begin to contract after cardioversion.

Digitalization, the usual medical treatment, slows the ventricular rate to provide adequate filling time and increases contractility for a better cardiac output. Other drugs that slow atrial activity are verapamil (Calan, Isoptin), quinidine, and propranolol (Inderal).

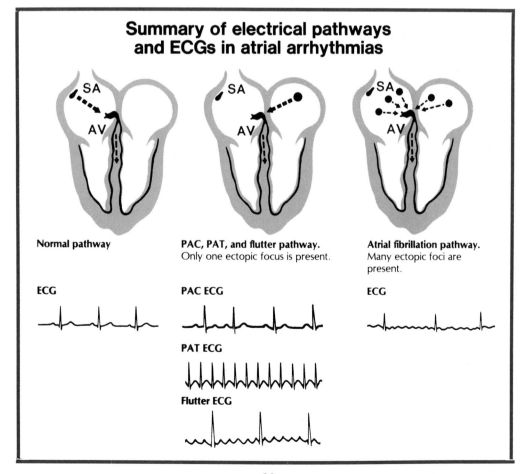

Summary of electrical pathways and ECGs in atrial arrhythmias

Normal pathway

PAC, PAT, and flutter pathway. Only one ectopic focus is present.

Atrial fibrillation pathway. Many ectopic foci are present.

ECG

PAC ECG

PAT ECG

Flutter ECG

ECG

Junctional (nodal) arrhythmias

After the cardiac impulse has traversed the atria, it reaches the atrioventricular junction (AV node). The AV node acts as a gateway to the conduction system that penetrates the dense muscular tissue of the ventricles. Its usual function is to receive the impulse, delay it for an instant, and then conduct it to the ventricular pathway. Junctional tissue in the area of the AV node also has the capacity to initiate impulses at the rate of 40–60 times per minute, and can act as a backup system if the sinus node fails to fire. In conditions of disease or anoxia, the tissue can become irritable and initiate rapid ectopic impulses.

Normal pathway　　　　　　　　**Junctional pathway**

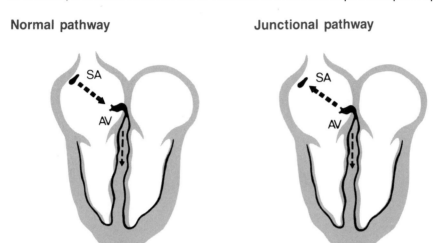

When an impulse arises in the junctional area, it will activate the atria through retrograde (backwards) conduction, causing the P wave to be inverted (in leads where the P would normally be upright). The impulse will be conducted through the ventricular pathways in a normal manner and thus the QRS will be normal.

The inverted P wave appears directly before, buried in, or directly after the QRS complex, depending on whether the atrium or the ventricle is activated first.

Junctional complexes

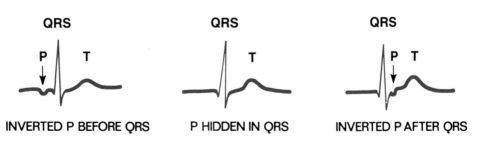

INVERTED P BEFORE QRS　　　P HIDDEN IN QRS　　　INVERTED P AFTER QRS

Junctional premature contraction (JPC)

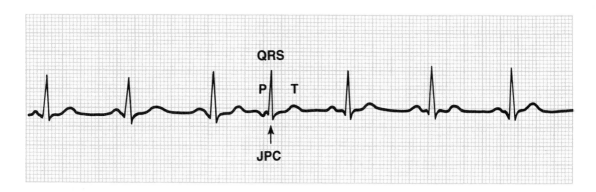

A **junctional premature contraction (JPC)** is an ectopic beat that arises from tissue in the junctional area and appears before the next expected sinus beat. The P will be inverted before or after the QRS, or it may be completely hidden in the QRS. The inverted P will always be very close to the QRS. A JPC can be distinguished from a PAC by the appearance of the P wave.

Infrequent JPCs do not require treatment. Frequent JPCs indicate tissue irritability and may be treated with a myocardial depressant.

Junctional rhythm

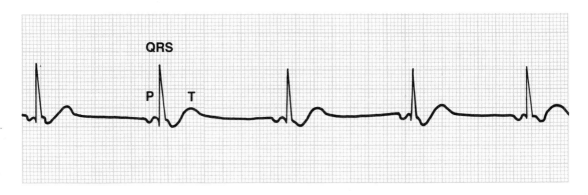

Junctional rhythm occurs when the pacemaker site is junctional tissue. The characteristic rate is 40–60 beats per minute, but this may be accelerated to the range of tachycardia. The rhythm will consist of repeated, regular junctional complexes.

Junctional rhythm may occur as a transient condition when the SA node is inadequate. It may also occur as a result of toxicity from digitalis or myocardial depressants. Treatment, if necessary, depends on the cause of the rhythm and the effect of the rate on the patient's clinical condition.

Junctional tachycardia

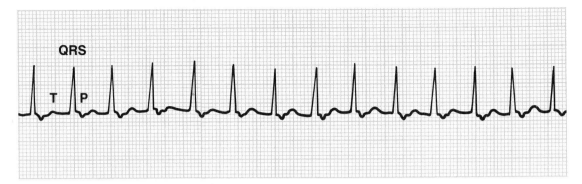

Junctional tachycardia is a junctional rhythm with a rate of 100–180 beats per minute.

This arrhythmia may be difficult to distinguish from sinus or atrial tachycardia. Whenever the origin of the tachycardia cannot be determined, and the QRS complex is of normal configuration, the term **supraventricular tachycardia** is used (often called SVT).

As with other fast-rate arrhythmias, this inefficient rhythm puts stress on the heart and may cause angina, congestive heart failure, or other dangerous conditions. Treatment would be similar to that used for atrial tachycardias. Digitalis toxicity may be a possible cause.

Wandering pacemaker

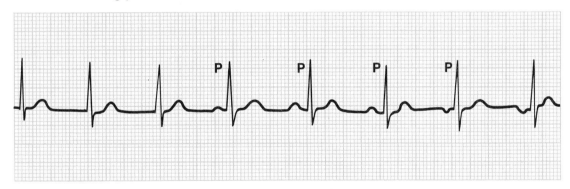

Wandering pacemaker is characterized by shifting sites of impulse formation, including the SA node and atrial and junctional tissue.

The P waves and PR interval may change from beat to beat depending on the pacemaker site. The rhythm is somewhat irregular. The QRS remains normal.

Wandering pacemaker will probably not produce symptoms; it may appear when there is no other evidence of cardiac disease. However, it may be associated with ischemia, inflammation, and digitalis effects. Usually, no treatment is necessary.

HOW TO READ AN ECG

PART IV

Ventricular arrhythmias

AV block

Artificial pacemaker

Ventricular arrhythmias

Ventricular tissue becomes more excitable as a result of ischemia, drug effect, or electrolyte imbalance. Arrhythmias originating in the ventricles may diminish the ability of the heart to function as a pump. Without adequate blood flow, all body organs deteriorate. Quick intervention is vital to correct certain ventricular arrhythmias.

Premature ventricular contractions (PVCs) or ventricular premature beats (VPBs) occur in most myocardial infarction patients and are the most common and easily recognized rhythm disturbances seen on the ECG. They are also seen in normal persons, and may be caused by smoking, coffee, or alcohol. When pathological, they are seen most often in patients with ischemic or arteriosclerotic heart disease.

Normal pathway	PVC pathways

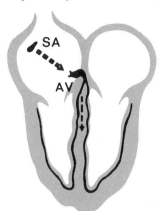 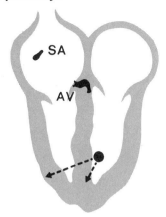

Normal and PVC pathways. As the name denotes, PVCs originate in the ventricles below the AV node. Because the PVCs do not follow the normal conduction path in the ventricles, they show a bizarre QRS configuration on the ECG.

ECG for PVCs

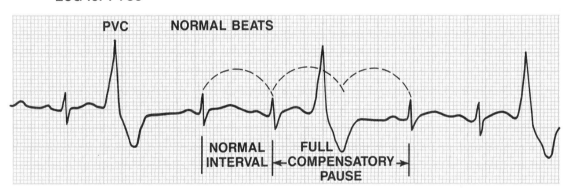

ECG for PVCs. Notice that the PVCs come early in the cycle (premature) and are wider than the normal beat.

Characteristics of PVCs

PVCs can be identified because they:
1. Usually occur early in the cycle.
2. Are not usually preceded by a P wave.
3. Have a wide and distorted QRS.
4. Have a large looping ST segment opposite in direction to that of the QRS.
5. Are usually followed by a full compensatory pause. (The interval between the R waves before and after the PVC is twice that of the normal R-R interval.)

Terms used to describe PVCs

Unifocal PVCs. Those that originate from the same site and therefore have the same configuration.

Multifocal PVCs. Those that originate from different sites and have different shapes.

ECG for multifocal PVCs

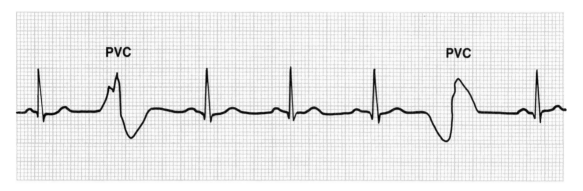

Bigeminy. Paired or coupled rhythm; a repeating pattern of two beats, with PVCs and normal beats alternating.

Trigeminy. Rhythm with a repeating pattern of three beats; the ratio of PVCs to normal beats is 2:1 or 1:2.

Interpolated PVCs. Those that fall between two normal beats without interrupting the rhythm. These PVCs are not followed by compensatory pauses.

ECG for interpolated PVC

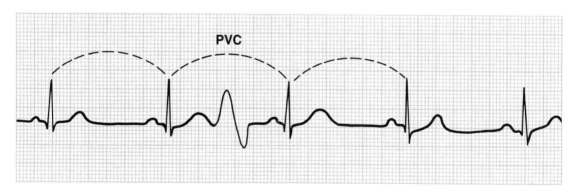

For the patient with an infarct, PVCs are usually given vigorous treatment because they can precipitate ventricular fibrillation by occurring on a T wave. They are especially dangerous when they:

1. Occur more frequently than one in 10 beats.
2. Occur in groups of two or three.
3. Are multifocal: Several ventricular sites are irritable.
4. Occur on or near the T wave. At this time (the vulnerable period) in the cycle, the conduction tissue is partially repolarized and may respond in an erratic manner. Some cells respond immediately and others later, causing intermittent depolarization and triggering ventricular fibrillation.

"Vigorous treatment" consists of giving lidocaine (Xylocaine), as outlined below in the section on ventricular tachycardia. When PVCs are seen with a sinus rate of over 60 per minute, lidocaine (a suppressant) is the drug of choice because the PVCs are most likely coming from an irritable focus such as ischemic tissue.

On the other hand, if sinus bradycardia occurs following a myocardial infarction, lidocaine may be contraindicated. Ventricular beats may be occurring as a compensatory mechanism to maintain a reasonable heart rate and provide some cardiac output. In this situation, atropine is given rather than lidocaine. It increases the rate of the slow-firing SA node and terminates the inefficient ectopic beats by replacing them with normal impulses. The usual treatment is 0.5–1.0 mg of atropine given IV.

Atropine is sometimes used in ventricular bigeminy with severe bradycardia for the same purpose: to speed up normal conduction and prevent re-entry beats from the ventricles.

Ventricular tachycardia. This dreaded complication of a myocardial infarction may be defined as a series of multiple (three or more), consecutive PVCs occurring at a rate usually between 150 and 200 per minute. Ventricular tachycardia is very dangerous because it leads to reduced cardiac output and, many times, to ventricular fibrillation.

Normal pathway

Ventricular tachycardia pathways

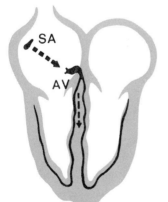
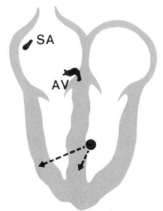

Normal and ventricular tachycardia pathways. These are the same sketches used to illustrate the PVC pathways since ventricular tachycardia can be

considered as a series of PVCs. Like the PVCs, the tachycardia shows a bizarre configuration on the ECG.

ECG for ventricular tachycardia

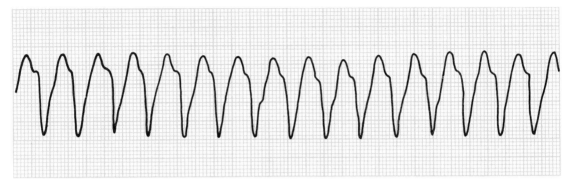

ECG for ventricular tachycardia. Notice that the rate is fast and that the QRS is wide. (A width of more than two and one-half small blocks is considered abnormal.) If the ventricular rate is not too fast, independent P waves may sometimes be visible in the QRS complex. (P waves are not seen in this example.)

Treatment of ventricular tachycardia. If the patient is tolerating this arrhythmia fairly well and has a pulse, IV lidocaine may be given as a bolus injection of 1 mg per kg of body weight followed by 0.5 mg per kg. If this is effective, a continuous IV drip of lidocaine should be started. Ventilation with oxygen is important. Procainamide hydrochloride (Pronestyl) may be given to patients who do not respond to lidocaine.

If drug therapy is ineffective and the patient becomes unconscious and pulseless, CPR and countershock should be instituted. Bretylium tosylate may also be used for recurrent or resistant ventricular tachycardia or fibrillation.

Torsade des pointes

Torsade des pointes (meaning turning on the points) is a form of ventricular tachycardia in which the QRS complexes change direction around the isoelectric line. Like ventricular tachycardia, it may stop spontaneously or progress to ventricular fibrillation. It usually does not respond to lidocaine.

Torsade des pointes occurs during a prolonged QT interval, which can occur from drug therapy, slow rate arrhythmias, electrolyte imbalance, and ischemic conditions. The cardiac drugs that can cause a prolonged QT interval include quinidine, procainamide (Pronestyl), disopyramide (Norpace), and amiodarone (Cordarone). The phenothiazides and tricyclic antidepressants may also trigger this tachycardia. It is desirable to monitor serum

levels of potassium, calcium, and magnesium during such drug therapy. Correcting deficiencies of these electrolytes may help to prevent or stop this dangerous arrhythmia. Bretylium tosylate and overdrive pacing are other possible treatments. Alertness for a prolonged QT interval is the most important aspect of prevention. The QT should not exceed one-half of the R–R interval.

ECG for Torsade des pointes

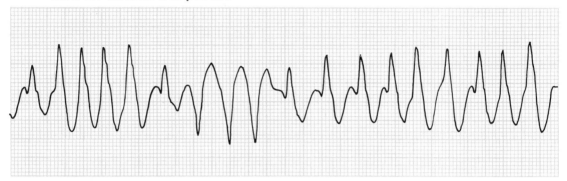

Ventricular fibrillation. It is extremely important to be cognizant of this rhythm; therapy should be instituted immediately. If the arrhythmia is not terminated, the patient will die within minutes.

Normal and ventricular fibrillation pathways. In the fibrillating heart, it can be considered that numerous ectopic foci in the ventricles are firing erratically. Thus, there is no effective contraction of the cardiac musculature, and the patient has no pulse.

Normal pathway

Ventricular fibrillation pathways

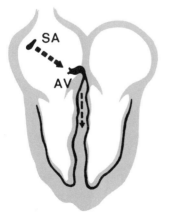

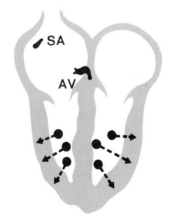

ECG for ventricular fibrillation

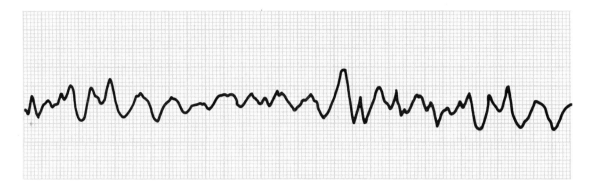

ECG for ventricular fibrillation. Notice the complete distortion and irregularity of the complexes. Since similar distortion may also be caused by the movement of the patient or the monitor wires, it is important to rule out these possibilities. If the patient is alert, or if not alert but has a pulse, the rhythm is **not** ventricular fibrillation.

PVC causing ventricular fibrillation

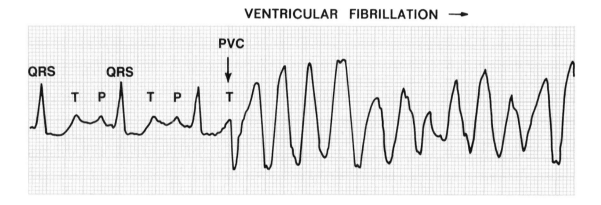

VENTRICULAR FIBRILLATION ⟶

PVC

QRS QRS

T P T P T

Treatment of ventricular fibrillation. If the patient is unresponsive and pulseless, call for help and begin cardiopulmonary resuscitation (CPR). At the onset of witnessed fibrillation, a precordial thump may be effective. If not, continue CPR and defibrillate as soon as possible starting with 200 joules.

Defibrillation depolarizes all of the myocardial cells simultaneously and allows the SA node to resume normal conduction. Be sure the synchronizer, which is used only for elective cardioversion, is turned off during defibrillation. If conversion does not occur after a third defibrillation attempt, IV drugs such as epinephrine, lidocaine, and bretylium tosylate may be given to increase contractility, perfuse the brain, and control ventricular excitability.

Good oxygenation of the patient with intubation and/or assisted respiration is vital to successful response and correction of acidosis. The use of sodium bicarbonate should be guided by blood gas results.

ECG of a successful defibrillation

VENTRICULAR FIBRILLATION   **ELECTRICAL DEFIBRILLATION**   **EFFECTIVE HEARTBEAT**

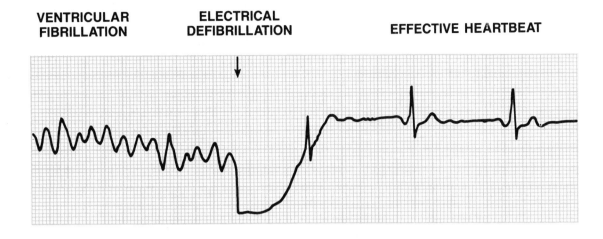

ECG of a successful defibrillation. Clearly shown is the point at which the electrical shock stopped the fibrillating heart. After a moment, the heart began to beat in normal fashion.

Patients who have frequent episodes of ventricular tachycardia and fibrillation not responsive to drug therapy are possible candidates for an automatic implantable cardioverter–defibrillator. AICD is a new electronic device that can monitor cardiac rhythm, detect ventricular tachycardia or fibrillation, and discharge a shock. The use of this device requires careful patient evaluation, extensive emotional support, and close monitoring for complications.

ECG for accelerated idioventricular rhythm

NORMAL BEAT   **FUSION BEAT**   **VENTRICULAR BEATS**

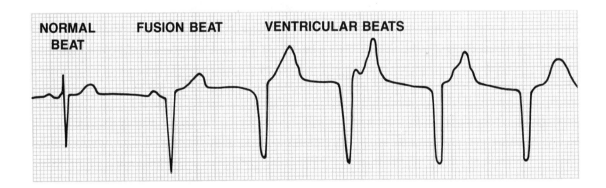

Accelerated idioventricular rhythm, "slow ventricular tachycardia," is another term used to indicate an arrhythmia originating from the ventricle. The rate is usually from 50 to 100. The QRS complexes are broad, and this rhythm may be preceded or followed by fusion beats. Accelerated idio-

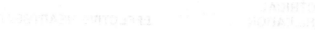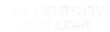

ventricular rhythm, which may occur in an acute MI, comes and goes spontaneously when the ventricular rate is close to the sinus rate. It may be a compensation for inadequate sinus function. It does not necessarily predispose to the development of ventricular tachycardia or fibrillation. Lidocaine is not used unless the rate changes to ventricular tachycardia. Assess the patient for inadequate sinus node function or possible digitalis toxicity as causes.

ECG for idioventricular rhythm

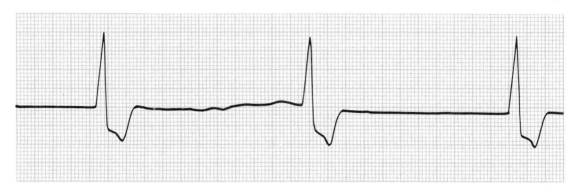

Idioventricular rhythm appears when all complexes originate from the ventricles (wide, distorted, identical QRSs). This occurs when there is no adequate atrial pacemaker, or when the impulse is blocked at the AV node. The rate corresponds to that of ventricular pacemakers (usually below 40).

The patient with this condition requires close observation and may be treated with stimulants and/or a pacemaker depending on the underlying pathology. When the ventricular function is due to clinical conditions that are not reversible, this is a terminal event. The complexes will gradually deteriorate to a straight line.

Ventricular standstill occurs when the ventricles do not respond to impulses from the atria. If this happens suddenly with complete heart block, only P

Ventricular standstill with complete heart block

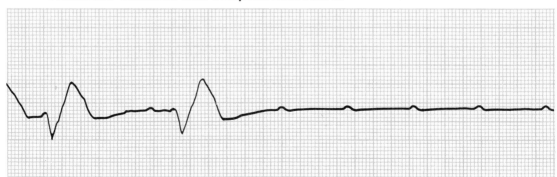

waves will be seen. No independent ventricular rhythm starts. The patient will have no pulse and CPR must be instituted immediately. Epinephrine IV and possibly atropine or isoproterenol (Isuprel) drip may help until pacing is started.

If there is no atrial activity and no compensating ventricular rhythm because of deterioration of tissue in both chambers, a secondary and terminal form of ventricular standstill may occur. There may be occasional electrical impulses without contractions.

Asystole. A sudden straight line on the monitor may be a mechanical problem or a patient problem. Check the patient first. If the patient does not respond, this may be a very fine line of ventricular fibrillation. Turn up the gain on the ECG monitor to check for this possibility. If fibrillation is present, defibrillate. If not, CPR and epinephrine would be indicated.

Electromechanical dissociation (EMD) Electromechanical dissociation occurs when myocardial cells depolarize but are unable to produce an effective contraction. An ECG pattern may appear. However, there is no pulse. Electromechanical dissociation may be secondary to another problem that diminishes cardiac function such as lack of oxygen or fluid volume, cardiac tamponade, tension pneumothorax, or pulmonary embolism. Treatment should be directed toward the perceived problem.

AV block

In this condition the AV node is diseased and has difficulty conducting the P waves into the ventricles. The most common causes are arteriosclerosis and myocardial infarction. Digitalis toxicity may also produce such blocks.

AV block

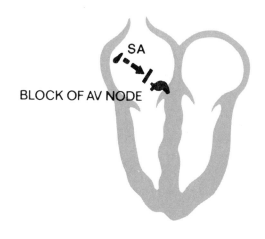

SA

BLOCK OF AV NODE

AV block. Scarring, inflammation, or edema prevents or slows transmission of the electrical impulse by the AV node. The degree of block varies from very slight to complete and is classified as first, second, or third degree block.

First degree AV block

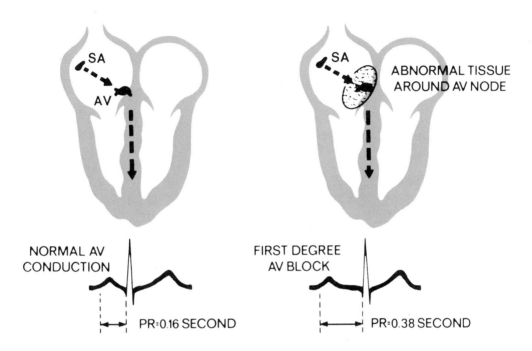

First degree AV block. Because the tissue around the AV node is abnormal, the impulse takes longer to traverse the area.

This is reflected by an increased length in the PR interval on the ECG. (The PR interval represents the impulse going through the atrium and the area of the AV node.) In contrast to second and third degree blocks, all P waves in first degree block penetrate the ventricles to form QRS complexes. In normal conduction, the PR interval is not over 0.20 second (five small blocks on the ECG paper where each block equals 0.04 second). A PR interval such as the one shown (0.38 second) is an indication of first degree block.

First degree block does not diminish cardiac output. However, it is an indicator of possible damage to junctional tissue or of drug effect, especially from digitalis. Careful observation is indicated for possible progression to higher degrees of block.

Second degree AV block exists when some of the P waves are conducted to the ventricles and others are blocked at the AV node. This condition is divided into two classifications: Mobitz I (Wenckebach) and Mobitz II, or Type I and Type II.

Mobitz I (Wenckebach) second degree block

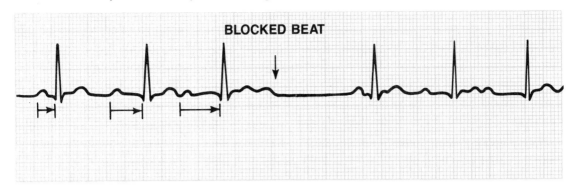

Mobitz I (Wenckebach). The ischemic or drug-affected AV node requires a progressively longer interval of time to transmit each beat until a beat fails to be conducted. When the next impulse arrives, the rested AV node is able to transmit the beat in a shorter time, but the PR interval again lengthens, and the cycle repeats.

On the ECG, this results in a progressive lengthening of the PR interval until a beat is blocked (P not followed by a QRS), and then the cycle repeats. The rhythm (R–R interval) is irregular, and there are more P waves than QRS complexes.

Wenckebach block may be caused by digitalis or MI, especially one involving the inferior wall. It is generally transient and reversible.

Observe the patient for an excessively slow ventricular rate. If treatment is required, atropine is the drug commonly used to speed the heart rate. Insertion of an artificial pacemaker generally is not necessary.

Mobitz II second degree block (2:1 ratio)

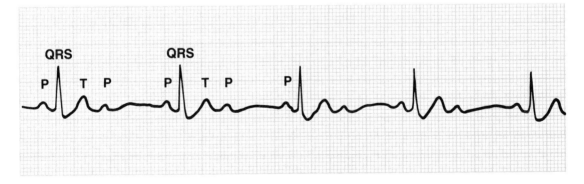

In **Mobitz II,** some beats are conducted and others are not. Conducted beats have a consistent PR interval. In blocked beats, there is a P wave not followed by a QRS complex.

One type of pattern shows a specific ratio of blocked beats such as 2:1, 3:1, or 4:1. In such cases, the R–R interval will be regular.

BLOCKED BEAT

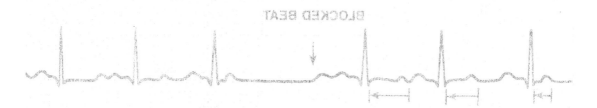

Mobitz I (Wenckebach). The ischemic or drug-affected AV node requires a progressively longer interval of time to transmit each beat until a beat fails to be conducted. When the next impulse arrives, the rested AV node is able to transmit the beat in a shorter time, but the PR interval again lengthens, and the cycle repeats.

On the ECG, this results in a progressive lengthening of the PR interval until a beat is blocked (P not followed by a QRS), and then the cycle repeats. The rhythm (R–R interval) is irregular, and there are more P waves than QRS complexes.

Wenckebach block may be caused by digitalis or MI, especially one involving the inferior wall. It is generally transient and reversible.

Observe the patient for an excessively slow ventricular rate. If treatment is required, atropine is the drug commonly used to speed the heart rate. Insertion of an artificial pacemaker generally is not necessary.

Mobitz II second degree block (2:1 ratio)

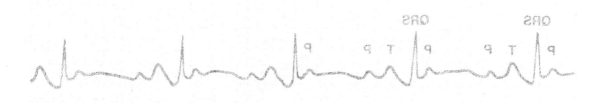

In **Mobitz II,** some beats are conducted and others are not. Conducted beats have a consistent PR interval. In blocked beats, there is a P wave not followed by a QRS complex.

One type of pattern shows a specific ratio of blocked beats such as 2:1, 3:1, or 4:1. In such cases, the R–R interval will be regular.

Mobitz II occasional blocked beat

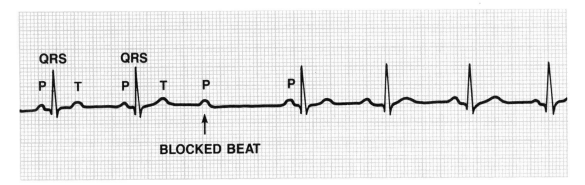

Mobitz II occasional blocked beat. Another pattern presents as an occasional nonconducted P wave. In this case, the blocked P will occur at the expected cycle interval.

One consequence of Mobitz II can be a slow ventricular rate resulting in low cardiac output. This diminished output can produce myocardial or cerebral ischemia. Early indications of cerebral insufficiency include restlessness, mental confusion, dullness, or agitation.

Mobitz II is more likely than Mobitz I to progress to a greater degree of block. Thus, to treat Mobitz II, many cardiologists insert a transvenous pacemaker that is activated when the cardiac rate falls.

To increase the heart rate while awaiting pacemaker insertion, 0.5–1.0 mg atropine IV may be given. If the rate cannot be maintained with atropine, an isoproterenol (Isuprel) 2–10 mcg/min drip may be infused. This is titrated for minimal rate needed until a pacemaker can be employed. The drip is cut back if ventricular irritability occurs.

Third degree AV block

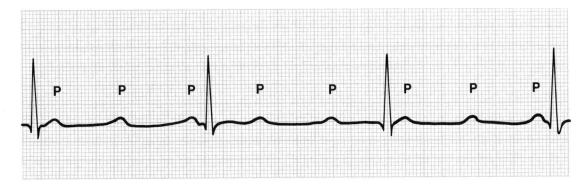

Third degree AV block is also called complete heart block. In this arrhythmia, no atrial impulses (P waves) activate the ventricles. The QRS originates from a junctional or ventricular pacemaker site. Therefore, the P waves and QRS complexes occur independently.

Both the P waves and QRS complexes occur regularly, but there is no relationship between them. The PR interval varies and some P waves may be partly obscured by QRS complexes.

Complete heart block may be caused by inflammation, scarring, myocardial infarction, or drugs such as digitalis. The pulse rate is usually slow because of the inherent rate of junctional or ventricular pacemaker sites. Since these secondary pacemakers are not dependable, the treatment of choice is an artificial pacemaker.

Atropine or, as a last resort, isoproterenol (Isuprel) may be given to increase the ventricular rate until a transvenous pacemaker can be inserted. During administration of isoproterenol, the monitor should be watched closely and isoproterenol stopped if frequent PVCs or ventricular tachycardia appears.

Conduction delays in AV blocks

AV block	Impulses	Rhythm	PR interval	ECG
First degree	All conducted (with delay)	Regular	Prolonged (>0.20 sec.); constant	
Second degree Mobitz I (Wenckebach)	Some conducted, some blocked	Irregular	Progressively longer until dropped beat; cyclic pattern	
Second degree Mobitz II	Some conducted, some blocked	Regular or irregular	Constant for conducted beats; some Ps without QRSs; can appear 2:1, 3:1, or occasionally blocked Ps	
Third degree	None conducted	Regular QRS; independent regular P	Variable; no P-QRS relationship	

Artificial pacemaker

An artificial pacemaker uses a pulse generator (power source) to stimulate the myocardium and produce a ventricular contraction. The power is delivered to the endocardium through a transvenous pacing catheter threaded into the right ventricle. Another way to stimulate the myocardium is through small electrodes sewn onto the surface of the heart, but this method requires a thoracotomy. An external pacing electrode system may be used for a short interval in an emergency situation.

A pacemaker may be indicated when sinus pacemaker activity malfunctions or the heart does not maintain a sufficiently rapid rate. Arrhythmias resulting in slow rates include sinus bradycardia or arrest that does not respond to drug therapy, heart block with a slow ventricular response, and bifascicular block with first degree block or trifascicular block.

Pacemakers are sometimes used to overdrive (capture and convert) fast-rate arrhythmias. This capability is called an antitachycardia function.

Prophylactic implantation may be done for patients with arrhythmias that may progress to inadequate rates during surgery, or when depressant drugs are being administered. Pacemakers may also be useful for stress testing in patients whose physical conditions contraindicate testing by the usual physical activity.

Transvenous pacemaker

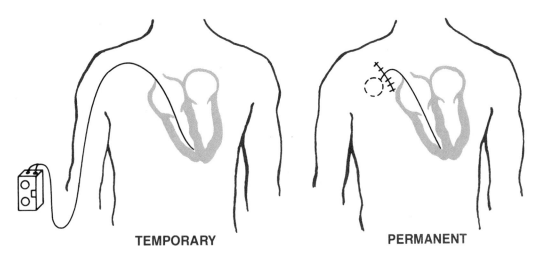

TEMPORARY   PERMANENT

A **temporary pacemaker** uses a transvenous catheter attached to an external pulse generator (power source). It can be inserted using fluoroscopy or ECG feedback for positioning.

For a **permanent pacemaker,** the pulse generator (enclosed in nonreactive material) is surgically implanted in superficial muscle tissue. The pacemaker function must be evaluated periodically and the unit replaced when necessary. Lithium batteries can last ten or more years.

The pacemaker artifact (blip or spike) is the ECG indication that an impulse has been fired. It appears as a vertical line above or below the baseline. If the electrode tip of the catheter is imbedded in functional ventricular tissue, the blip will be followed immediately by a wide QRS (similar to a beat originating in the ventricle). Pacemaker stimulation of the atrium will appear as a blip followed by a P wave. A pacing artifact is not produced by the heart's natural activity and will continue even if the electrode tip is out of place or the patient has expired.

A **fixed-rate** (asynchronous) pacemaker is not designed to sense the patient's natural beat and fires at a constant, preset rate. It is useful only when the patient has no spontaneous ventricular contraction.

Continuously functioning artificial ventricular pacemaker

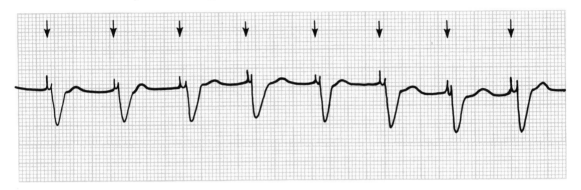

Continuously functioning artificial pacemaker. The ECG shows a small vertical line (see arrows) at the beginning of each QRS complex. This line represents the electrical stimulus of the artificial pacemaker.

Demand pacemaker

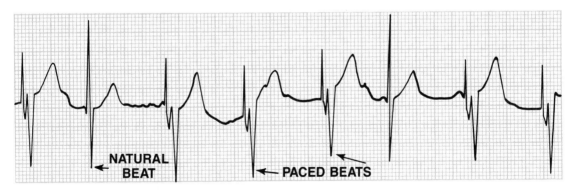

The **demand pacemaker** discharges only if the pacemaker does not sense a natural impulse within a preset time interval. Demand pacing avoids competition between paced and natural beats. A demand pacemaker is used to maintain a minimum rate (for example 64 to 78) and does not limit faster natural rates.

A **synchronized pacemaker** that relays the patient's atrial impulse to the ventricle provides the benefits of a physiologically variable rate.

An **atrioventricular sequential pacemaker** triggers first the atrium and then the ventricles to provide the added cardiac output from atrial contraction. Different modes, as seen on the dual chamber pacemaker, allow for one or both chambers to be sensed and paced.

A **programmable pacemaker** can be adjusted by noninvasive means after the pacemaker is implanted. Variables may include rate, output, pacing mode, and sensitivity. Reprogramming, which is done by the physician through magnetic switches, can produce changes to meet the patient's needs.

Classification of pacemakers

In order to assess pacemaker function, it is necessary to know what the pacemaker can and should do. Because of the increasing complexity of pacemaker information, the Inter-Society Commission for Heart Disease suggested a standardized letter coding system. The original (1974) three-letter code described the functional capabilities of pacemakers including chamber paced, chamber sensed, and mode of response. The code was revised in 1981 to include programmable functions and tachyarrhythmia functions.

For example, a ventricular demand pacemaker that senses and paces the ventricles to maintain a set rate is classified as VVI. The I indicates that ventricular stimulus is inhibited when a spontaneous ventricular beat is sensed.

Chamber(s) paced	Chamber(s) sensed	Mode of responses (sensing function)	Programmable functions	Special tachyar-rhythmia functions
1974				
V = Ventricle	V = Ventricle	T = Triggered		
A = Atrium	A = Atrium	I = Inhibited		
D = Double (dual)	D = Double (dual)	(demand)		
	O = None	O = None (continuous)		
1981				
V = Ventricle	V = Ventricle	T = Triggered	P = Programmable	B = Bursts
A = Atrium	A = Atrium	I = Inhibited	M = Multiprogrammable	N = Normal rate competition (dual demand)
D = Double (dual)	D = Double (dual)	(demand)		
	O = None	D = Double (dual function: T and I)	O = None (Permanent pacemakers only)	S = Scanning
		O = None (continuous)		E = External
		R = Reverse		

Pacemaker problems

A systematic approach to pacing problems will reduce confusion and result in a more rapid identification of the difficulty. Begin by checking the patient, including symptoms and vital signs. If the patient is unstable, report to the physician immediately and initiate emergency measures as indicated. After stabilizing the patient, determine why the pacemaker was originally inserted. Obtain a rhythm strip; if the tracing does not show the pacing blip clearly, check the ECG from another lead. Find out the type of pacemaker to understand its capability and expected function.

Pacemaker problems can occur because a pacing electrode becomes displaced or because of mechanical failure, which can involve the wires, battery, or electrical circuits.

Non-capture (no contact between pacemaker and heart)

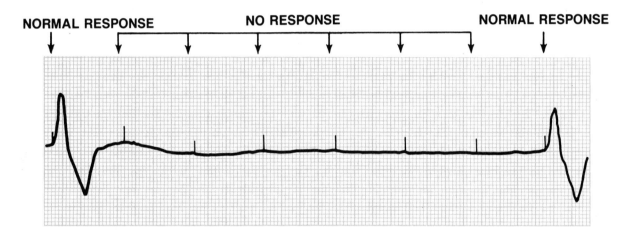

NORMAL RESPONSE   NO RESPONSE   NORMAL RESPONSE

Non-capture (no contact between pacemaker and the heart muscle). This is one of the most common causes of pacing failure. It occurs when the catheter wires pull loose from the heart wall or are in contact with an area of nonresponsive scar tissue. It is readily identified in the ECG. The QRS complex that normally follows the pacemaker stimulus (left arrow at top of example) suddenly disappears. It resumes (right) when contact is made again. Notice that the small vertical line of the pacemaker stimulus continues, indicating that the pacemaker is functioning but does not result in contraction of the heart muscle. Capture may be improved by having the patient cough or turn. To provide the necessary rate, the voltage may be increased on a temporary external pulse generator until the catheter can be repositioned by the physician.

Competition occurs when a pacemaker fails to sense the patient's natural beat and fires on top of it. Competition is especially dangerous when the artificial pacing impulse occurs during the vulnerable period of the cardiac

cycle (the T wave). A stimulus at this time may cause a disorganized rhythm such as ventricular fibrillation.

Failure to sense can be caused by poor contact of the electrode tip or from mechanical problems of the wire or battery. Initial measures to correct the problem include increasing the sensitivity of a temporary pacemaker, replacing battery, and repositioning the patient. If these measures are ineffective, a more sensitive temporary pulse generator should be used.

When **pacemaker failure** occurs, the patient will be dependent on the heart's natural ability. This can result in decreased cardiac output. Support the patient's hemodynamic needs and prepare to initiate pacemaker repositioning or replacement as necessary.

Pacemaker stimulation of the diaphragm will result in hiccups. This can occur because of excessive pacemaker voltage or perforation of the heart muscle by the lead. Reposition the patient and check the voltage. It may be necessary to surgically reposition the wire.

As pacemaker complexity increases, the possibilities of pacemaker malfunction also become more complex. For example, some of the dual-chambered programmable pacemakers can initiate impulses that re-enter conduction pathways and cause tachyarrhythmias. These mechanisms are similar to those causing arrhythmias naturally. All problems that do not respond to simple troubleshooting measures must immediately be referred to an experienced physician for diagnosis and treatment.

HOW TO READ AN ECG

PART V

Miscellaneous rhythm disturbances;
Blocked PAC

Aberrancy

Bundle branch block

Fusion, capture, and escape beats

AV dissociation

Wolff-Parkinson-White syndrome

Effects of drugs and electrolytes on the ECG

Miscellaneous rhythm disturbances

This section contains definitions and brief descriptions of more complex rhythm disturbances that may confuse interpretation in ECG monitoring. Additional information about these subjects can be found in comprehensive electrocardiography textbooks.

ECG for blocked PAC

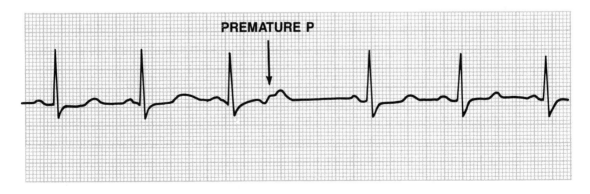

PREMATURE P

Blocked premature atrial contraction (PAC). A blocked PAC occurs when an irritable focus in the atria fires a premature impulse that depolarizes atrial tissue; the impulse is not conducted to the ventricles. The P wave occurs before the T wave of the preceding beat is completed.

At this early point in the cycle, the AV node and ventricular tissue are refractory (cannot respond) because they have not yet been repolarized following the previous beat. On the ECG, this appears as a premature P wave not followed by a QRS complex.

Note that the P wave (sometimes buried in the T wave of the previous beat) is premature. It is important to differentiate this blocked PAC from the Mobitz II, which shows an occasional blocked beat (P not premature), and from sinus arrest (no P). The most common reason for a pause in sinus rhythm is a blocked PAC. Blocked PACs may be present in normal hearts, or may occur because of digitalis toxicity or heart disease. A blocked PAC is harmless but the blocked beat of Mobitz II may warn of AV nodal damage.

An aberrant beat is one that is initiated by the SA node and then deviates from normal conduction in the ventricles. Intraventricular conduction defect (IVCD) is a general term sometimes used to describe this phenomenon. It implies a block in one of the bundle branches.

The term aberrancy is most likely to be used when trying to differentiate the origin of beats characterized by a wide, bizarre QRS complex. Such beats may originate from the ventricles (ectopy) or from sinus/atrial tissue acquiring the wide QRS as a result of the deviant ventricular pathway (aberrancy). Determining the correct origin is significant because ectopic beats are more dangerous than aberrant beats.

Bundle branch block is an obstruction in the right or left ventricular conduction pathway. When this occurs, the impulse travels first through the unobstructed branch and is then transmitted by nonspecialized myocardial tissue to the opposite ventricle. This aberrant pathway requires a longer time for activation of the ventricles, and the resulting QRS is greater than 0.12 sec (three small squares). Origin of this beat is from the atria—usually, the SA node. Therefore, a P wave will precede the wide QRS.

Bundle branch block may occur in a single premature beat, because either the right or left branch has not yet been repolarized. It may occur when the rate becomes too fast to permit adequate repolarization between beats (rate-dependent). It may also result from disease or ischemia in this part of the conduction system.

To determine which bundle branch is blocked, we must look at lead V_1 or modified chest lead I (MCL$_1$). From this viewpoint on the right side of the heart, we can observe the direction of current flow.

When the **right bundle branch** is blocked, the impulse travels first through the left ventricle (upward deflection or R wave), and then activates the right ventricle (second upward deflection or R'). This produces an M-shaped complex in V_1 or MCL$_1$.

If the entire **left bundle branch** is blocked, the impulse first depolarizes the right side of the heart and then—through aberrant pathways—the left ventricle, producing a wide, deep V-shaped complex. A small, upright R may appear before this complex.

Right bundle branch block

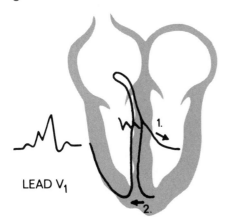

LEAD V₁

Left bundle branch block

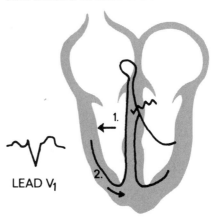

LEAD V₁

Right bundle branch block is more common because the right branch is a long, narrow pathway. The left bundle branch is thicker at its origin and subdivides into anterior and posterior branches. When one of these subdivisions (fascicles) becomes blocked, it is called a hemiblock, or monofascicular block. It does not produce a QRS greater than 0.12 sec, and is diagnosed by axis determination. When the right bundle branch and either fascicle of the left bundle become blocked, it is called bifascicular block.

Trifascicular block indicates a combination of two "fascicles" plus first degree AV block. This is dangerous because of the many areas involved, and a pacemaker is indicated.

Conduction pathway-hemiblock

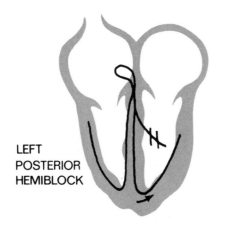

LEFT
POSTERIOR
HEMIBLOCK

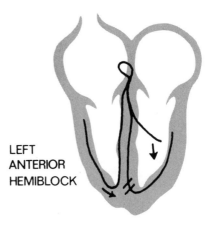

LEFT
ANTERIOR
HEMIBLOCK

Bundle branch block can occur in healthy hearts and in a variety of disease conditions. Additional data are required to determine its significance. Cardiac depressant drugs should be used with caution because they can aggravate the conduction delay.

Fusion, capture, and escape beats occur as a result of variations in timing of impulses.

ECG for fusion beat

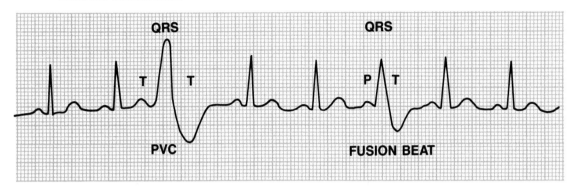

A **fusion beat** results when an impulse from the sinus node activates the atria just when an ectopic ventricular impulse discharges. This coincidence produces a P wave before a wide QRS complex in which the QRS is partly normal and partly like a ventricular beat.

A fusion beat may appear as a single beat, or it may initiate a run of ventricular beats or ventricular tachycardia. The fusion beat will occur late in the cycle after a P wave that arrived at the normal cycle interval. This can be differentiated from a PAC with aberrant conduction (a wide QRS because the PAC occurred so early that a bundle branch was not yet repolarized and therefore was refractory). In the PAC, the P wave will occur earlier than the usual P–P cycle interval. Fusion beats are dangerous and should be treated with lidocaine. Aberrant PACs are not dangerous.

ECG for capture beat

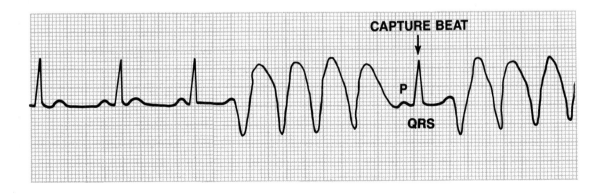

A **capture beat** is an impulse that takes control of the heartbeat. For example: A ventricular capture beat is conducted from another area to "capture" the ventricles.

During an episode of ventricular tachycardia, the atria continue to function independently. Occasionally, an atrial impulse occurs when the ventricles can respond. This one beat, conducted through the ventricles in a normal fashion, results in a normal complex in the midst of a run of ventricular tachycardia.

The significance of seeing such a beat is that it proves the other beats are really ventricular tachycardia and not atrial tachycardia with aberrancy. This is often difficult to differentiate. When there is doubt, treatment is based on the patient's clinical needs.

Capture also refers to an ectopic pacemaker (a VPC or JPC "capturing" the atria), or to a beat generated by an artificial pacemaker.

ECG for escape beat (junctional)

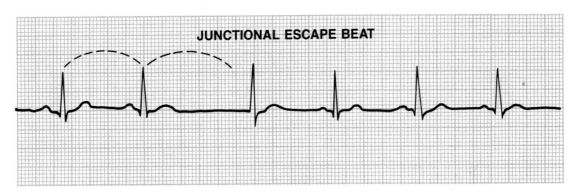

JUNCTIONAL ESCAPE BEAT

An **escape beat** may occur after a pause longer than the usual R–R interval. It originates in junctional or ventricular tissue and functions as part of the heart's backup pacing system to prevent cardiac arrest. It compensates for a lapse in sinus node activity. If a conducted rhythm does not resume, this escape beat may initiate a continuing rhythm.

ECG for AV dissociation–accelerated junctional rhythm coexisting with sinus beats

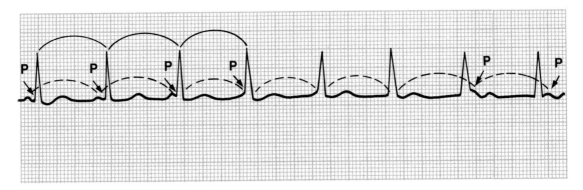

AV dissociation exists whenever separate pacemakers simultaneously control the atria and ventricles. Two separate sites send impulses, and independent rhythms coexist to pace the upper and lower chambers.

The term AV dissociation is used by different authors to describe a variety of conduction disturbances. The following are some of the more widely recognized variations:

AV dissociation can exist because of an inadequate atrial pacemaker. For example: When impulses from the sinus node or atria are excessively slow, pacemakers from the junctional or ventricular areas interpose escape beats or rhythms.

When the atrial pacemaker impulse is intermittently blocked from the ventricles, separate atrial and junctional or ventricular rhythms may be established. These rhythms may have almost identical rates.

Irritability in an ectopic site may result in a rapid junctional or ventricular rhythm. A separate atrial rhythm coexists—for example, ventricular tachycardia with unrelated P waves.

Digitalis toxicity may be the cause of many such rhythms as it slows normal conduction and increases the automaticity of secondary pacemaker cells.

ECG for Wolff-Parkinson-White (WPW)

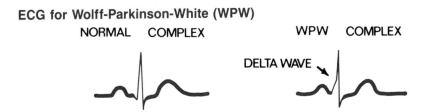

NORMAL COMPLEX   WPW COMPLEX

DELTA WAVE

Wolff-Parkinson-White (WPW) syndrome. A pre-excitation syndrome exists when atrial impulses are transmitted directly to the ventricles through shortcut conduction pathways. The impulses do not travel through the AV node and thus avoid the normal conduction delay that occurs there.

The syndrome carries the names of the physicians who described one atypical conduction pattern. The ECG is characterized by:

1. A short PR interval (less than 0.12 sec)
2. A slurred upstroke on the QRS (delta wave)
3. A wide QRS (greater than 0.10 sec)
4. Secondary ST and T wave changes (repolarization is altered)

The mechanism of WPW is thought to be the utilization of a highly developed accessory branch of the conduction system called the bundle of Kent. This connects the conduction system of the atria to either ventricle, bypassing the AV node. This could occur on either the left (type A) or right (type B) side of the heart. Impulses go down the accessory pathway and return by the normal conduction system to set up a re-entry system.

Patients with this condition are subject to episodes of supraventricular tachycardia. This arrhythmia may be resistant to the usual treatment for PAT.

It is important to differentiate it from ventricular tachycardia and other arrhythmias with wide QRS complexes.

Another pre-excitation pattern is the Lown-Ganong-Levine syndrome, characterized by a short PR interval without a delta wave.

Effect of drugs and electrolytes on the ECG. Changes in ECG configuration may result from the presence or absence of certain substances that influence myocardial tissue. Here are the most common, listed with their ECG effects:

Agent	Effect on myocardium	ECG change	Example
Hypokalemia (low serum potassium)	Increases irritability (ectopic beats) (v. tach.)	Decreases height of T wave; produces U wave; prolongs Q–T	
Hyperkalemia (high serum potassium)	Depresses automaticity (standstill)	Creates tall, peaked T waves; prolongs PR interval; shortens Q–T	
Hypocalcemia (low serum calcium)	Decreases threshold for stimulation (v. tach.)	Prolongs Q–T interval	
Hypercalcemia (high serum calcium)	Increases threshold for stimulation	Shortens Q–T interval	
Digitalis	Depresses conduction; increases automaticity (predisposes to many arrhythmias)	Produces downward deflection of ST segment; prolongs PR interval	
Quinidine	Depresses conduction and automaticity; may cause 1:1 conduction in atrial flutter (v. tach.)	Widens QRS; prolongs PR interval; prolongs Q–T	

Many additional drugs, such as antiarrhythmics and tranquilizers, can change the ECG pattern. Drugs need not reach toxic blood levels to produce ECG changes.

REVIEW QUIZ

Review questions are provided so that you can check your understanding of the information presented in the text. The questions are arranged by chapter and answers are supplied at the end of the section.

Part I. Questions (Monitoring)

1. Electrocardiographic monitoring provides information about the heart's
    a. coronary arteries
    b. force of contraction
    c. electrical activity
    d. cardiac output

2. When the monitor shows a straight line, you should begin troubleshooting by checking the
    a. attachment of the lead wire
    b. patient
    c. on-off switch
    d. lead selector switch

3. Which patient is at highest risk for electrical hazards? A patient with:
    a. telemetry
    b. Holter monitor
    c. arrhythmias
    d. a temporary pacemaker

4. Which is most likely to cause false low-rate alarms?
    a. gain set too low
    b. gain set too high
    c. electrodes placed over bony protuberances
    d. patient movement

5. A method for transmitting electrocardiographic signals by radio waves is
    a. computerized monitoring
    b. telemetry
    c. Holter monitor
    d. portable monitor-defibrillator units

6. Which finding is *LEAST* likely to indicate cardiovascular compromise?
    a. headache
    b. restlessness
    c. decreased urinary output
    d. reduced BP

7. **Which of these electrodes is always negative?**
   a. left leg
   b. left arm
   c. right leg
   d. right arm

8. **Poor electrode contact can cause**
   a. wandering baseline
   b. intermittent loss of signal
   c. false low rate alarms
   d. all of the above

9. **Whenever there is a change in the ECG rhythm during continuous monitoring, you should first:**
   a. notify the physician
   b. reset the low-rate alarm
   c. evaluate the effect on the patient
   d. reposition the electrodes

10. **After the cardiac impulse leaves the SA node and depolarizes the atria, it goes to the:**
   a. Purkinje fibers
   b. left bundle branch
   c. AV node
   d. bundle of His

Part II. Questions

1. **The normal physiological pacemaker is the:**
   a. bundle of His
   b. AV node
   c. SA node
   d. Purkinje fibers

2. **The normal PR interval is**
   a. 0.10–0.12
   b. 0.12–0.20
   c. 0.04–0.12
   d. 0.04–0.20

3. **The wave form that represents ventricular repolarization is the:**
   a. P
   b. PR
   c. QRS
   d. T

4. **A fresh myocardial infarction is characterized on the ECG by:**
   a. rate changes
   b. rhythm changes
   c. ST elevation and T wave inversion
   d. ST depression and T wave elevation

5. **Lead II shows electrical activity from the:**
   a. right arm to left leg
   b. right arm to right leg
   c. left arm to left leg
   d. left arm to right leg

6. **Whenever electricity flows from a negative pole toward a positive pole, it causes a deflection that is:**
   a. upward
   b. downward
   c. both upward and downward
   d. isoelectric

7. **The SA node normally discharges at the rate of:**
   a. 40–60
   b. 60–80
   c. 20–40
   d. 60–100

8. **On the ECG, the P wave corresponds to:**
   a. atrial depolarization
   b. ventricular depolarization
   c. ventricular repolarization
   d. junctional repolarization

9. **On the ECG paper, the width of each small square is:**
   a. 0.02 sec
   b. 0.04 sec
   c. 0.12 sec
   d. 0.20 sec

10. **The definitive ECG sign of a transmural infarction is:**
    a. a prominent Q wave
    b. tall T waves
    c. ST elevation
    d. wide QRS

Part III. Questions (Supraventricular rhythms)

1.

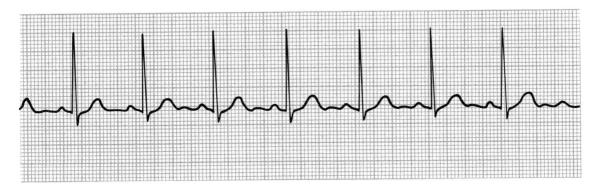

    a. Is the rhythm regular?
    b. What is the rate?   Is this normal?
    c. Do P waves occur at regular intervals?
    d. What is the PR interval?   Is it the same for all beats?
    e. Interpretation?

2.

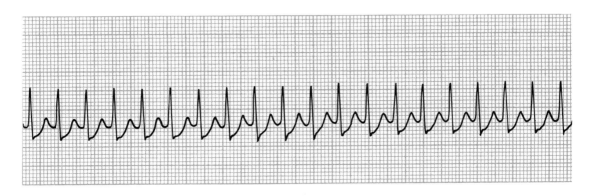

    a. What is the rate?   Is the rhythm regular?
    b. Are there P waves before each QRS?
    c. Where might they be?
    d. Interpretation?
    e. Is there any potential problem from this rhythm?
    f. What is the usual treatment?
    g. Are there other possible drugs/measures that might be useful?

3.

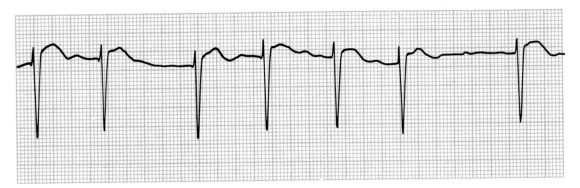

    a. Is the rhythm regular?
    b. What is the rate?
    c. Are P waves clearly discernible?
    d. Interpretation?
    e. Does this rhythm decrease cardiac output?   Why?
    f. What is the usual medical treatment?

Part IV. Questions (Ventricular and conduction disturbances)

1.

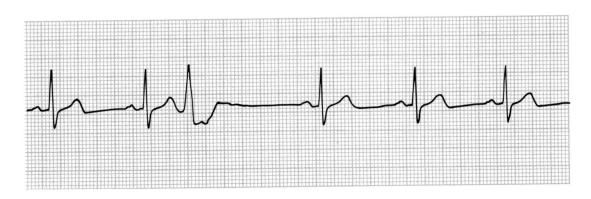

    a. Is the rhythm regular?
    b. Are there P waves before all QRS complexes?
    c. Are all QRS complexes normal?
    d. Interpretation?
    e. Is there any potential danger?
    f. What is the usual treatment?

2.

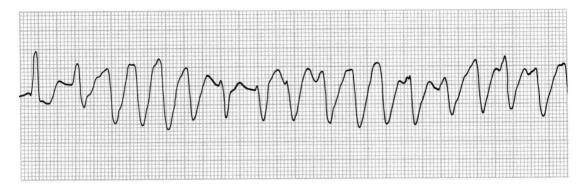

    a. Are there P waves before all QRS complexes?
    b. Are the QRS complexes normal?
    c. Interpretation?
    d. Is the sinus node in control of the heart?
    e. Is this dangerous?   Why?
    f. What is the usual medical treatment?

3.

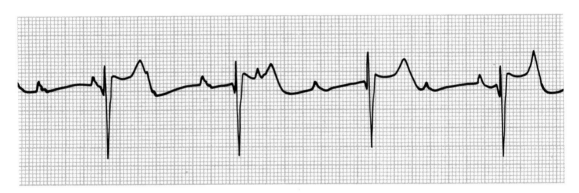

    a. Is this rhythm regular?   What is the rate?
    b. Do P waves occur at regular intervals before the QRS?
    c. Is there a relationship between the P wave and the QRS?
    d. Are atrial impulses being conducted to the ventricles?
    e. Is this dangerous?
    f. What is the usual treatment?
    g. What might help until this is accomplished?

Part V. Questions (Miscellaneous rhythm disturbances)

1. **In a blocked PAC, the P wave is:**
   a. absent
   b. premature
   c. at the expected time
   d. delayed

2. **Whenever separate pacemakers simultaneously control the atria and ventricles, this is called:**
   a. trifascicular block
   b. WPW syndrome
   c. AV dissociation
   d. bundle branch block

3. **This beat occurs after a pause that is longer than the usual R–R interval:**
   a. fusion beat
   b. capture beat
   c. escape beat
   d. blocked PAC

4. **What ECG changes might be seen in the patient who is taking digitalis?**
   a. downward deflection of ST, prolonged PR
   b. wide QRS, shortened PR
   c. prolonged Q–T interval
   d. tall, peaked T waves

5. **In which of these conditions should you notify the physician and prepare for possible pacemaker insertion?**
   a. right bundle branch block
   b. frequent blocked PACs
   c. left hemiblock
   d. trifascicular block

6. **Individuals with Wolff-Parkinson-White syndrome are subject to episodes of:**
   a. atrial tachycardia
   b. ventricular tachycardia
   c. sinus bradycardia
   d. third degree block

7. **Which ECG features would you look for in the patient who has hypokalemia?**
    a. tall, peaked T waves, prolonged PR
    b. decreased height of T wave, U wave present
    c. absent P waves
    d. wide QRS

8. **When one beat is conducted normally in the midst of a run of ventricular tachycardia, this beat is called a/an:**
    a. escape beat
    b. capture beat
    c. aberrant beat
    d. fusion beat

9. **A wide, M-shaped QRS complex in V_1 or MCL_1 may indicate:**
    a. right bundle branch block
    b. left bundle branch block
    c. anterior hemiblock
    d. posterior hemiblock

10. **A beat characterized by a short PR, a slurred upstroke on the QRS, and a wide QRS is:**
    a. a blocked PAC
    b. a fusion beat
    c. bundle branch block
    d. WPW syndrome

Answers to Quiz

I. 1. c   2. b   3. d   4. a   5. b
     6. a   7. d   8. d   9. c   10. c

II. 1. c   2. b   3. d   4. c   5. a
     6. a   7. d   8. a   9. b   10. a

III. 1. a. yes   b. 75, yes   c. yes   d. 0.18 sec, yes
     e. normal sinus rhythm
     2. a. 187–190, yes   b. hidden   c. buried
     in the preceding T   d. atrial tachycardia
     or SVT   e. decreased cardiac output
     f. vagal stimulation, cough, or Valsalva
     maneuver   g. Verapamil, Tensilon,
     Inderal, or possibly elective cardioversion

3. a. no   b. ventricular rate 70   c. no
d. atrial fibrillation   e. yes, loss of atrial
component to filling   f. Digitalis

IV. 1. a. yes except for one premature beat
b. all except the premature beat c. premature beat is wide, others are normal
d. sinus rhythm with PVC   e. ventricular irritability could progress to ventricular tachycardia or fibrillation.   f. IV Lidocaine if PVCs are frequent, or patient has
other cardiac instability
2. a. no   b. no   c. ventricular tachycardia   d. no   e. yes, could progress
to ventricular fibrillation   f. Lidocaine
bolus and drip
3. a. yes, ventricular rate 43; atrial rate
100   b. no   c. no, PR intervals
change   d. no   e. yes, secondary
pacemakers are not dependable and
the rate is too slow   f. artificial
pacemaker   g. Atropine or Isuprel

V. 1. b   2. c   3. c   4. a   5. d
    6. a   7. b   8. b   9. a   10. d

Determining heart rate

Large Squares:			**1**					**2**					**3**					
Small Squares:	3	4	5	6	7	8	9	10	11	12	13	14	15	16	17	18	19
Rate:	500	375	300	250	214	187	167	150	136	125	115	107	100	94	88	83	79

Large Squares:	**4**					**5**					**6**					**7**		
Small Squares:	20	21	22	23	24	25	26	27	28	29	30	31	32	33	34	35	36
Rate:	75	71	68	65	62	60	58	56	54	52	50	48	47	45	44	43	42

Large Squares:			**8**					**9**					**10**					
Small Squares:	37	38	39	40	41	42	43	44	45	46	47	48	49	50	51	52	53
Rate:	41	40	39	38	37	36	35	34	33	33	32	31	31	30	30	29	28

Count the number of small or large squares on the ECG paper between two con-secutive R or P waves and use this table to determine the precise heart rate (beats per minute), provided the rhythm is regular.

DATE DUE

JAN 0 1 1998		
MAY 1 0 2001		
APR 0 4 2003		

Demco, Inc. 38-293